MY FATHER'S BRAIN

MY FATHER'S BRAIN

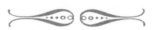

Life in the Shadow
of Alzheimer's

SANDEEP JAUHAR

Farrar, Straus and Giroux
New York

Farrar, Straus and Giroux
120 Broadway, New York 10271

Printed in the United States of America
First edition, 2023

Library of Congress Cataloging-in-Publication Data
Names: Jauhar, Sandeep, 1968– author.
Title: My father's brain : life in the shadow of Alzheimer's / Sandeep Jauhar.
Description: First edition. | New York : Farrar, Straus and Giroux, 2023. |
    Includes bibliographical references and index.
Identifiers: LCCN 2022055023 | ISBN 9780374605841 (hardcover)
Subjects: MESH: Jauhar, Prem P. | Alzheimer Disease | Father-Child Relations |
    Personal Narrative
Classification: LCC RC523 | NLM WT 155 | DDC 616.8/311—dc23/eng/20221223
LC record available at https://lccn.loc.gov/2022055023

Our books may be purchased in bulk for promotional, educational, or business
use. Please contact your local bookseller or the Macmillan Corporate and
Premium Sales Department at 1-800-221-7945, extension 5442, or by email at
MacmillanSpecialMarkets@macmillan.com.

www.fsgbooks.com
www.twitter.com/fsgbooks • www.facebook.com/fsgbooks

1   3   5   7   9   10   8   6   4   2

The names of some persons described in this book have been changed. In some
places the order of events has been changed for the sake of narrative cohesion.

For Rajiv and Suneeta

Be kind to your father, even if his mind fails him.

—SIRACH 3:13

Life without memory is no life at all.

—LUIS BUÑUEL

CONTENTS

CONTENTS

PART II: SCARS

MY FATHER'S BRAIN

INTRODUCTION: THEY USED TO CALL ME TOPPER

We were sitting in the waiting room of the same neurology practice that was treating my mother's Parkinson's disease when my father asked me, perhaps for the third time, "Why am I here?"

"Because your memory is getting worse," I answered.

"My memory is fine," he replied. Any lapses, he had been insisting, were normal for a man of his age.

"So what did you have for lunch?" I asked, staring ahead.

He thought for a moment, then sniffed defiantly as my point came across. "Well, no one can remember everything," he muttered.

He and my mother had moved to Long Island, where my brother and I lived, several months earlier. Since their arrival, I had come to suspect that his symptoms were not the usual age-related cognitive changes, even if he kept saying they were. For example, he had always been careful with his money, a consequence of an impoverished childhood, but now he was bouncing checks. He was booking hotel and flight reservations but neglecting to cancel them—something my older brother, Rajiv, discovered only after he began to monitor my father's bank accounts. Nearly every week he was sending cash to random charities in response to generic emailed or televised appeals.

"Two fifty here, a hundred there," Rajiv said. "Not that much, but I'm not sure he knows what he's doing." When we voiced our concerns, my father said it was his money and that he would spend it the way he wanted.

So, despite nearly four decades of medical experience between us, my brother and I decided our father needed the attention of a specialist. As cardiologists, we understood diseases of the heart. My father's problems, we realized, were on a different plane.

For his part, my father seemed unconcerned. Memory loss, to him, was an inevitable consequence of aging. In the sixth century B.C., the Greek philosopher Pythagoras of Samos divided the life cycle into five distinct stages, the last two of which he designated the senium, a period of decline and decay of the human body and mental faculties "to which, very fortunately, few of the human species arrive, [as] the system returns to the imbecility of the first epoch of infancy." In his casual fatalism, Pythagoras had a fellow traveler in my father.

I had been asking him, "How do you think your memory is?"— foolishly hoping that if he could at least recognize the problem, he might try harder to overcome it.

"My memory is fine," he would say.

"But you are always forgetting things."

"Everybody forgets, Son," he would assure me. "It happens with everyone."

The irony here was that my father had once hated the prospect of losing his faculties, even when there was little reason for him to fear such a thing. I remember standing in Riverside Park on a wintry day about ten years earlier, when I was still living in New York City, yelling at him on the phone for stopping his blood pressure medications again. Though a respected scientist, he had never trusted drugs (or doctors) to keep him well.

"Do you want to end up with a stroke?" I blared into the phone after he told me his systolic blood pressure was still hovering around

160 or higher (greater than 140 is considered hypertension) on the rare occasions that he checked it. "You won't be able to work."

"I'd rather be dead," he replied, before agreeing to restart the medications.

Yet now here he was, sitting amid vinyl chairs and potted plants, nonchalantly sipping free coffee from the Keurig machine as we sat and waited for his name to be called. He asked me, again, how he could become an organ donor. Once again, I gave him the response he did not want to hear: that because of his advanced age, the options were limited.

"Come on, Sandeep," he implored. "I have wonderful organs!"

"We'll look into it," I said, not wanting to discuss his organs in the waiting room.

"Just tell me where I can get a donor card." He stood up, picking up his briefcase. "I will ask here."

"Sit down," I hissed as people began to stare. "You can't tell random people you want to donate your organs. Like you asked that lady at the front desk, 'Do you know any widows I can give money to?'"

"I didn't."

"You did! That is not how things work. You have to go through the proper channels."

"You are not telling me the proper channels."

"Fine, so we'll look it up. But Dad, come on, you're seventy-six years old."

Obviously disappointed, he began to say something, but then we heard his name, Prem Jauhar, called out. I quickly stood up and patted him on the shoulder to follow me. Dr. Marc Gordon was ready to see us.

I had first recognized something was amiss only four months earlier, when I'd flown to North Dakota, where my parents then lived, to attend my father's retirement party.

My parents lived in a development of brick homes, square lawns, and young trees about ten miles from the Fargo airport. Pulling up to their house that scalding July afternoon, I immediately noticed a "For Sale" sign on the front lawn. But the swing set for the grandchildren was broken, and my mother's prized garden was overrun with weeds. Walking up the front steps, I saw oil stains on the driveway and rust on the garage girders. The house did not look like it belonged on the market.

My parents were in the living room when I arrived. Though she was growing increasingly frail, my mother, Raj, insisted on standing up to hug me. She had been suffering from Parkinson's disease for several years by then, and her movements were jerky and slow. Still, she looked beautiful in a yellow silk salwar kameez and gold bangles, her hair specially dyed with henna for the occasion. My father's hair was whiter and more flyaway than I remembered from the last time I had seen him about a year before. He looked like he had lost some weight, too. "Hi, Bubboo," he said affectionately, patting me on the head as though I was eight years old again. Then, before I could hug him, he turned to my brother-in-law—my sister, Suneeta's, husband, Vini—who had arrived a few minutes earlier, and said, "As I was saying, Vini, life is hell here. It was the worst winter we have ever had."

I had not been at my parents' home since the previous summer, but I observed right away that most of the house did not appear lived in. Soap dispensers were empty and lightbulbs needed to be replaced. A bottle of Drakkar Noir cologne, a gift no doubt from my brother, was sitting on my father's bedside table unopened. Inside the closet that served as my mother's shrine, brass bowls, usually filled with incense ash, had been wiped clean. The usual litter of burnt matches, signifying prayer, was nowhere to be seen.

In the basement, hard-shell Samsonite suitcases were stacked in a corner, along with some old board games, old shoes, and old books that remained to be packed. My mother's shawl hung on a nail, amid rumpled sweaters and my father's cheap print shirts.

I went into my father's study. Hanging on the wall was a framed plaque he had received at a farewell luncheon in his honor a few months earlier. "We are made strong by difficulties we face and do not evade," it said. Black-and-white electron micrographs were spread over the desk, and the filing cabinets were still loaded with his papers. I opened the drawers and thumbed through hanging folders, looking for something, though I wasn't sure what. I came across the usual files: "Intergenomic chromosome pairing in wheat," "Cytological characterization of trigeneric hybrids." I found several copies of an old issue of the Fargo-Moorhead *Forum* with a picture of my smiling father under the headline "NDSU Geneticist Creates Scab-resistant Wheat."

Then I came across a folder labeled "Dementia." Inside it was an article printed from CNN.com with the title "Dementia After Retirement: How to Delay or Avoid." It had obviously been read many times because recommendations like "learn a new language," "take enough steps," and "stay socially active" were underlined in different colors of ink.

"What are you doing?"

I jumped. My father was standing in the doorway. "Nothing," I said, quickly putting away the folder. I scanned the desk and pointed to a black-and-white photograph of my father in college. He was standing tall, posing with his friends, a stark contrast to the old man waiting impatiently at the door. "I've never seen this picture," I said.

"Leave it," my father said. "We have to go to the party."

"Were those your college friends?"

"Yes," he said. "They used to call me Topper. Because I was always at the top."

I laughed. "You look so young. You can't be more than sixteen."

"I was in second grade before the partition of India," he said. "The teacher said I was too smart, so when we resettled, they put me in the fourth grade."

I closed the drawer, my heartbeat speeding up. "Dad, I think that was me. I was the one who skipped two grades, remember? You met with the principal in Kentucky."

"I skipped those grades, too," he said after a short pause.

"The same grades? Are you sure?"

"Yes," he said. "Now, come on. We must leave for the party."

At Dr. Gordon's office, a medical assistant took us into a chilly exam room with a computer, a small desk, and three chairs. A poster on the wall depicted a decaying autumn tableau: a fogged-over pond lined with tangles of bare trees and fallen red leaves. The assistant pulled a fresh sheet of paper onto the vinyl examination table and asked my father to sit on it. He did so agreeably, making a quip about how he was still a young man. Then, with an automated cuff, she checked his blood pressure. She put two fingers on his wrist and counted his pulse. She checked his temperature and weight. All vital signs were normal.

After a few minutes, Dr. Gordon came in. Curly-haired and bespectacled, dressed in rumpled khakis, a checkered blue shirt, and a mismatched tie, he looked every bit a practitioner of the intellectual specialty to which he belonged. I had run into him a few times recently at the hospital and briefed him on my father's condition; he had suggested bringing my father in for neurocognitive testing. Gordon now shook my father's hand warmly. "How are you, Dr. Jauhar?" he said.

"Fine," my father replied quickly. "Everything is fine."

Gordon took a seat at his workstation and started tapping on the keyboard. At this initial visit, many fields in the electronic medical record needed to be filled in, so I took the lead in answering Gordon's questions. Fortunately, my father was physically healthy. He was on a baby aspirin and medications (at least sporadically) for blood pressure and cholesterol, but he had no serious medical problems and had had no significant hospitalizations. My father sat quietly as I spoke. Perhaps he was tired, I thought—he usually napped in the early afternoon—or had forgotten some details, or maybe he felt cowed by Gordon's authority. Or possibly, I wondered, glancing at him sitting stiffly, hands on his lap, his shirt pocket thick with a wallet and a few pens, he knew something was wrong, even if he kept denying it, and was relieved that his problems were finally getting the attention of a specialist.

I told Gordon that we first noticed my father's memory trouble after he moved to Long Island three months earlier, in August. In the beginning it seemed benign enough. He would forget the names of old acquaintances. He could not remember the four-digit combination to his new safe. But soon the lapses became more concerning. At family get-togethers, he would tell the same story over and over. He would point to photographs and ask me to identify people, ostensibly as a test of *my* memory of our family history. There were long-forgotten aunts and uncles—but in some cases my own infant children! It was a startling transformation. He was a world-class scientist, had been running a wheat genetics lab up until a few months before, and was a fellow of the American Association for the Advancement of Science.

"And the American Society of Agronomy," my father added.

"That, too," I acknowledged before continuing to detail his memory problems.

He had been living with my mother in the community of Hicksville for almost three months, yet routes he should have learned in that time were still not committed to memory. He had gotten lost driving home from Walgreen's, which was only a mile away. He must have thought he was at the CVS across the street because he exited right out of the parking lot instead of left, circling for almost two hours in unfamiliar neighborhoods before stopping the car to ask a stranger for directions. His cognitive troubles were affecting his mood, too. He was frequently becoming enraged, a big change for him. He had recently pushed my mother's home health aide during an argument.

"What are you saying?" my father erupted.

"We have to talk about these things, Doctor," Gordon interjected. "Your son wants me to understand what your troubles are, so he has to describe some things that I am asking him. If you disagree, of course, please tell me."

But for the remainder of this portion of the interview, my father was silent.

When he turned to my father, Gordon spoke with the agreeable, if slightly patronizing, tone of a senior physician. My father was cooperative enough while answering Gordon's questions, though I could tell he found some of them demeaning. Of course he knew the date (November 12, 2014), though not the place (Manhasset). (Not a big deal, I told myself; he had had few occasions to come out this way.) He remembered events from my childhood—even his own childhood—but recent events were fuzzy. He did not remember a recent party at his house or what he had had for lunch that day. "Does it bother you that you don't remember some things, Doctor?" Gordon asked.

"You can't remember everything," my father replied, eliciting a chuckle from the neurologist.

The physical examination was normal. My father's sensation, coordination, motor strength, and reflexes were equal and symmetric. But on a cognitive test called the mini-mental state examination, there were some slipups. He started off all right. He was able to count backward from one hundred by sevens, and he properly named a watch, keys, and a pen. He knew recent news about the Islamic State, and he remembered the words "spinach," "violin," and "elephant" immediately after they were spoken and then again after about three minutes. When asked to write a sentence, he wrote, "You're a nice man."

However, he made some unexpected mistakes. He spelled the word "world" correctly forward but not backward ("D, L, O, R, W"). He said the president was George Bush before correcting his answer to Barack Obama. He also had difficulty drawing a clock with the time eleven ten. Inexplicably he forgot there were hour and minute hands and that the marks for three and nine should be perpendicular to twelve and six. This, I would later learn, is a telltale sign of impaired visuospatial reasoning. "It is not correct," my father said as he handed the drawing back to Gordon.

"Why not?" Gordon asked.

"I did not go into the details," my father explained.

"Why not, Doctor?" Gordon pressed.

"Because I didn't want to," my father snapped.

When the exam was finished, Gordon explained his findings. My father had scored 23 or 25 points out of 30 on the mini-mental test, depending on how Gordon decided to score a couple of the answers. This result, buttressed by the history I had provided (and the one my father had been unable to provide), was consistent with a diagnosis of mild cognitive impairment (MCI) of the "amnestic" type.

The term "MCI" was actually new to me. In nearly two decades in medicine, I had never heard of it. The diagnosis first appeared in the psychiatric literature in 1988, but it has roots in earlier papers going back to the 1960s in which it is referred to as "mild dementia," "limited dementia," "questionable dementia," and "senescent forgetfulness." MCI, Gordon explained, meant that my father's cognitive functioning was worse than expected for his age, but probably not bad enough to be classified as true dementia. Though there were measurable deficits in several mental domains, most notably memory, my father was still able to compensate for them so that most people meeting him would not know that something was wrong. However, as with most patients who have the condition, he was beginning to require some assistance with more complex activities, such as driving.

MCI, Gordon said, affects up to one in five elderly adults. Twenty percent of those affected by MCI, maybe more, will go on to develop full-blown dementia (Gordon speculated my father might already be at an early stage). There were some things—like eating a healthy diet, exercising regularly, and taking part in social events—that my father could do to decrease the odds. But there was no way to predict the course of the disease. We could do further testing, Gordon told us, such as a special PET scan looking for beta-amyloid, an abnormal protein that accumulates in the brains of Alzheimer's patients. But the scan was expensive, insurance wasn't going to pay for it, the presence (or absence) of beta-amyloid correlated only weakly with disease activity, and there were no good treatments for Alzheimer's anyhow, so Gordon said he would not recommend it. This did not surprise me. Though often master diagnosticians, neurologists usually have depressingly little to offer their patients.

Nevertheless, Gordon said he was going to start my father on Aricept, one of four drugs approved for Alzheimer's. Treating dementia with Aricept is a bit like using Tylenol for arthritis. The drug might improve my father's memory (however minimally), but it would do nothing to slow the progression of his cognitive impairment. Still, Gordon said, if my father could remain at the level he was, that would be a small victory. He recommended bringing him back for a follow-up visit in six months.

"Thank you for your time, sir," my father said as we got up to leave, seemingly oblivious to the life-changing news that had been delivered. He asked Gordon for his business card and then offered his own, a simple yellow card printed with his name, his address, and the title "Fellow of the AAAS." At the bottom were the words "Success is a journey, not a destination."

When we got back to my car, I opened the door for my father, and he got into the front passenger's seat. He struggled with the seatbelt for a few seconds before giving up and asking me to clip it in. I got behind the wheel and backed out, deep in thought.

"So, what did the neurologist say?" my father asked as we waited at a stoplight.

"He said you are having memory problems."

My father scoffed, turning to stare out the window. "But that is normal at my age, isn't it?"

It was my mother who first asked that we take my father to a neurologist. We had gone for a walk in their Hicksville neighborhood one breezy fall evening. Birds were chirping, sprinklers were going, children were riding tricycles on an otherwise empty street. My mother had been telling me how my father had gotten lost driving home from Sears the previous weekend. Though she had instructed him to call one of the children, he had decided instead to stop the car on the main road and flag down passersby for directions. As I helped her up the steps into the house that September evening, she turned to me and finally whispered the question we had all been afraid to ask: "Does your father have Alzheimer's?"

Lewis Thomas, the physician and essayist, called dementia, of which Alzheimer's is the most common type, "the worst of all diseases." No doubt my mother would have agreed. To her, the loss of control and social stigma, the eventual total dependency and need for institutional care, were the worst possible fate in old age—worse, even, than the Parkinson's that had robbed her of her motor function and the life she had enjoyed.

When we moved to the United States in 1977, the country was in the midst of what could be called the "Great Alzheimer's Awakening." Research conducted earlier in the decade suggested that the disease, far from being rare, as was previously thought, was actually one of the leading causes of death in American society—on par with heart disease and cancer.

Since that time, as more and more of us survive into old age, that finding has taken on the texture of an incontrovertible fact. Today, everybody knows someone with dementia. The number of American adults estimated to have Alzheimer's or related dementias has reached 6 million today—about one in every ten Americans over the age of sixty-five—and is projected to double in thirty years. At the midpoint of this century, the condition is expected to afflict almost 15 million Americans and more than 100 million people worldwide, likely eclipsing cancer as the second most common pathway to death (heart disease remains the first). In polls, dementia is actually more feared than cancer. It is more feared than death itself.

The visit to Dr. Gordon that fall of 2014 set our family off on a journey. Over the next several years, we would cope with my father's deterioration while I set off on my own quest to understand his brain and the brains of other patients afflicted with dementia. This book is an account of that journey. It is about my relationship with my father, especially during the last phase of his life, as he succumbed to his disease. It is also about the complications that arise when family members must become caregivers, the bonds of siblings, and the testing of those bonds. Though the conversations and conflicts are personal, they are also in many ways universal—icons of conversations and conflicts that every family facing the mental erosion of an elder has. In addition to this personal story, the book is also about the brain and how and why it degenerates with age, how memory gives meaning to our lives, even as it falters or changes with time, how dementia complicates our understanding of what it means to be a person—and what all this means for patients, their families, and society at large.

The knowledge I gained helped me to enter my father's world. It helped me to bridge—if only partly—the gap between us, one I had struggled to cross, in one way or another, my whole life. Still, it was probably the hardest journey I have ever taken. For nearly seven years I pushed and prodded, threatened and cajoled, begged and pleaded, encouraged and ridiculed. I made my father walk, bought him books, forced him to do puzzles. I loved him, cared for him, and hated him, too.

"Don't forget me," his eyes seemed to say. So, as a son, I endeavored to keep my memory of him intact. I eventually came to know more about him—who he was, his likes and dislikes—than he knew about himself. That was a strange responsibility to carry. At gatherings I would find myself saying, "He wrote books. He won academic prizes." I was reminding everyone that he was more than his disease.

Eventually I could only remember him in pieces. My middle-aged memory was failing me, too. I would have visions of him in his younger days. Hints of his old self would appear in words and gestures—vague, distant, like a feeling, barely etched—but sometimes the elements would coalesce, and then there he was, my erstwhile father, pulling me along to the bus stop in my starched white school uniform, squeezing my fingers tightly, as I now squeezed his. My memory was a figment, of course, and yet that figment seemed like less of a ghost than the man he had become.

As we drove away from Dr. Gordon's office that chilly November day, I did not know the details of what lay ahead. But as a physician, I knew that the disease was going to win in the end. There would be no surprises, no miracles; the battle would be lost. The only question in my mind was how much was going to be sacrificed in the defeat.

PART I

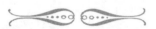

OF PLAQUES
AND
TANGLES

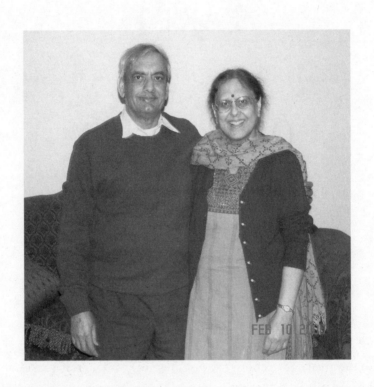

WE COULD ALWAYS MOVE TO GEORGIA

One morning in July 2014, about a week before I flew to Fargo for my father's retirement party, I received a troubling email from his former neighbor. Though I had met the neighbor a few times—I had even reached out to invite him to the party—he still felt compelled to introduce himself.

"I am Ajit Damle," he wrote. "I used to live in Fargo, across the street from your parents. I retired from the local hospital as a cardio-vascular surgeon recently and now have moved to Florida.

"I have known Prem and Raj ever since they landed in Fargo. It is with the greatest affection that we remember them. Prem's unassuming manner (till you get to know him!) hides his extraordinary status as a world-class scientist. As we became friends over the years, I came to admire his character more and more. Raj is so loving; even for a casual knock-on-the-door visit, she never let us out without feeding us her delectable Punjabi cooking. Over time they both were elevated to the senior patriarchal status in the local Indian community.

"Unfortunately we will not be able to attend on July 19, but I will call and write to Prem and Raj. I am glad they are moving to New York, and I saw on my last visit that the house was for sale. Just so you know, I advised Prem occasionally re: financial planning and some other advice. I was very concerned that he is not what he used to be. Forgive me if I am frank, but my respect and fondness for Raj and Prem makes me write so."

The email continued: "Your parents recently visited with us in Tampa. We had a frank discussion about how they would survive post-retirement. They were visibly anxious. They told me about their finances, and I do not think they have anything to worry about. But that needs some planning.

"I know you all love them dearly and will look after them self-lessly. However, now that I am 63 and retired, I understand better the geriatric psychology. The natural fallback position for them is mild paranoia, and they will (like any in-laws) not want to rely on your spouses. So if you can convince them to go to a financial planner and a lawyer for wills, etc., it will serve them well. They want to live independently but are not sure how."

Living independently in their old age was the last thing my parents had ever planned to do. In the culture they had left behind when they emigrated from India nearly four decades earlier, sons (or, rather, their wives) were supposed to take care of aging parents. In a country with no safety net to speak of, adult sons were the most reliable form of social security. So, well before we could voice an opinion on the matter, it was already assumed that when the time came, my parents would live with either Rajiv or me. "We cleaned your bottoms when you were babies," my father often reminded us. He did not need to spell out that he expected repayment in kind. What would happen to my parents when they could no longer care for themselves was a heavy subject, laden as it was with my parents' anxieties not only about their well-being and security, but also about their children's cultural choices and whether their parental authority would fade as we matured. It was no laughing matter. The only time I remember my father kidding with us about it was when he asked if Rajiv and

I would give him free medical care in his old age. I assured him that we would give him a discount.

But over the years, as my brother, sister, and I moved away and the family unit fragmented, my parents' blueprint for old age faded into an extracted promise that they were reluctant to redeem. The shift began during our teenage years, when my brother and I clashed with them over dating, drinking, and other rites of passage of American culture, but it continued as we moved on to college and medical school and carved out independent existences. Hewing to a plan hatched in the shadow of an India that itself had changed was not going to be easy—for us or for our parents. None of us wanted to live under the same roof again. If my parents were too traditional for us, we were too modern for them.

Still, even if it was rarely discussed, the question remained: Where would my parents live when they could no longer live independently? We put off talking about it, as most families do, until my mother's diagnosis with Parkinson's disease in 2011, about twenty years after we had all left the family home, lent some urgency to the situation. As her condition deteriorated, my brother and I pressed my father to retire and move with my mother to Long Island to live closer to us. He was not ready to do that, however. He had just reached the top of the U.S. Department of Agriculture pay scale as a full professor at North Dakota State University and wanted to reap some financial rewards for all his years of hard work.

Then, in 2012, my father told me his department had instituted a rule requiring faculty members to publish at least two research papers a year. It was an arbitrary standard, surely designed to force out aging scientists like my father, yet one I believed he could easily meet; he had already published more than a hundred peer-reviewed papers in the world's most prestigious scientific journals. But strangely, my father began to say that he believed his days in academia were numbered. He told me he did not want to produce low-quality papers under deadline that would mar his stellar record. He began to spend increasing amounts of time at the office trying to get the work done, though seemingly making little progress. In retrospect I should have known that if my father was worried that he could not meet his own high standards, things were worse than they appeared.

Thus began a series of uncomfortable conversations in which my father tried to gauge my brother's and my sincerity in asking him and my mother to move to Long Island to live near us. "We could always move to Georgia," he would say passive-aggressively to my mother. "I hear Athens is nice." (My parents knew no one in Georgia.) We tried to allay his concerns—Rajiv even offered to buy them a house on Long Island—though my father's persistent insecurity about his standing in our lives is what gave us pause about pushing the move in the first place. If they had been less traditional, my parents probably would have chosen to move to Minneapolis to live near my younger sister, Suneeta, and her family. But their culture would not allow them to rely on a daughter and a son-in-law in their old age.

In the end, after nearly two years of unresolved discussions, my father finally announced in November 2013 that he would be retiring in the summer of 2014 and that he and my mother would be moving to Hicksville, a small town on Long Island about eight miles equidistant from Rajiv and me. It was also where my mother's cousin Nani lived. With its Hindu temples and dosa shops, Hicksville could hardly have been more different culturally from the predominantly white Midwestern community my parents had lived in for the past twenty-five years. My father said that they were moving closer to family because of my mother's illness. But by then, I suspect, the relocation was maybe for him, too.

In August, then, my parents moved into a two-bedroom, split-level home on a quiet Long Island street in the kind of homespun neighborhood in which they had spent the better part of their lives in America, though this one was considerably more diverse. For nearly forty years, they had lived in America with their feet firmly planted in the India of their memories, leaning over to peer into their new world but never really embracing it. Now that they were finally living around people with whom they had more in common, at least culturally, we were hoping that they would feel comfortable in their final years.

But when they arrived on Long Island, I was alarmed by how much my parents' conditions had deteriorated, even since my visit to Fargo the previous month. My father was touchy and forgetful; my mother required assistance with walking. To help manage the move, they had brought Sharon, their good-natured cleaning lady, with them for two weeks. Stout, sturdy, and bespectacled, the product of three generations of Fargoans of northern European stock, Sharon had known my parents for many years and so, like a bar magnet picking up iron filings, was able to make quick order of the nearly two decades' worth of clutter they had transported with them. One evening, while arranging cutlery in the kitchen, she took me aside. "Things are sliding," she said bluntly. I thought she meant my mother, but it was actually my father she was more worried about.

"His mind gets confused sometimes, like things are all swirling up in there and he can't keep it all straight," she said. "I worry how he's going to take care of himself, let alone take care of your mother. He has to have everything settled one, two, three, or he gets confused." Earlier that summer, she told me, he had gotten lost driving home from his lab in Fargo. She had been at the house when he called, so she directed him back.

"Another time he called me over there," she said, as I listened quietly. "He says, 'I'm putting my house up for sale, what do I need to do?' 'Well, we have to make the house look presentable,' I say. 'Don't jump the gun.' He says, 'When do I need to book my tickets?' I say, 'You've moved before, Prem, across continents even. Don't tell me you don't know how to move.' He says, 'Last time, the government moved for me. I don't know how to do this.' I knew he was worried, and that your mom wasn't going to be able to do it, so that's why I came."

She added, "If he's slipped so much in a year, I worry about what's going to happen next."

On Long Island, with near-daily contact, my father's decline was even more obvious to me than it had been in Fargo. For a man who usually insisted on having his way, he seemed curiously aloof during the move-in. He had little to say about where to place the furniture or the televisions or what to put up on the walls. He did insist, however, on hanging up a poster that read "Happy Birthday" and listed the names of each of his grandchildren. "It will save time," he explained.

In Fargo, his schedule had been strict and regimented, but now his days seemed shapeless. Every afternoon, and even most mornings, he would take a nap, drawing the curtains, rather than running the air conditioner, to keep out the rancid heat. When he wasn't napping, he would watch television, mostly Indian soap operas and Bollywood music videos.

This was especially peculiar because at one time he had been a news junkie. On the Sunday mornings of my childhood, the voice of David Brinkley was as familiar as my mother's urging us to come to the table for her potato parathas. When I was in middle school, my father and I would go to the library at the University of California at Riverside, near where I grew up, to read *The New York Times* or books and newsmagazines on politics and foreign policy—especially nuclear arms control, which was a special interest of mine. For my thirteenth birthday, he gave me a book of famous front pages from the *Los Ange-*

les Times: "Peace," "Walk on Moon," "Nixon Quits." Later, we always watched *Nightline* together after the rest of the family went to bed. He had always encouraged his children to keep up with the events of the world. But now it was dance videos 24-7, along with the saccharine ads for Prem Jyotish, astrologer and numerologist, offering his phone services at five dollars a minute.

I thought I could engage my father by asking about his research, but now that he was retired, it seemed to hold little interest for him. I hired a college student to help him with his memoirs, which he had been planning to write for a number of years, but she stopped coming after he kept canceling their appointments.

Then, one morning, as sunlight streamed through the small kitchen window, he asked me why he was taking only six medications per day. "What will I take on the seventh day?" he wanted to know.

At first, I convinced myself that the lapses were a consequence of the stress of retirement and moving and the loss of a familiar routine. Things would get better, I told myself, as my father got more comfortable in his new home and made new friends. So we made sure to invite Nani, my mother's cousin, and her husband, Omi, to our family gatherings, hoping they would introduce my parents to their social circle. But they remained cool and distant, perhaps aware of where things were heading and reluctant to assume more responsibility than they could handle.

For forty-nine years my parents had done almost everything together, and so maybe it was fitting that my mother would be sliding, too. In Fargo she had barely been able to stand up on her own. Now, her physical disability was even more striking. On nights when I would visit after work, she would be sitting at the dining table among my father's strewn papers, spilling food on her bib. Once quick to smile, her face now appeared expressionless. Conversations, once so easy with her, stopped flowing. Parkinson's caused dangerous drops in her blood pressure, too, resulting in frequent falls. She had even stopped cooking. In Fargo, Sharon told me, my parents had been eating cereal for dinner three times a week. Living two thousand miles away, we hadn't known.

Her deterioration no doubt was hard on my father; the physical work required to care for her was itself overwhelming. She resisted using a bedside commode, so he was constantly walking her to the bathroom, even in the middle of the night, when we feared she would fall and break a hip. He would wake up at six in the morning to administer her thyroid medicine, then again at nine o'clock to give her the rest of her pills. Each morning he would make her walk on a treadmill, despite the fact that she was increasingly off-balance. He would lose his temper if the part-time aide we had hired prematurely terminated the exercise, even if it was at my mother's insistence. "You have little concern for my wife," he would hiss.

His anger would boil over at my mother's rotating cast of aides, especially when they would begin their shifts in the morning after a sleepless night for him. He would say he did not need them, that they were a waste of money, that he could manage on his own. Some were too "modern" or "independent" for him. One he accused of "showing off." I would explain to them that my father was not in his right mind. Needing work, most would put up with the abuse. Even so, we went through seven aides in the span of two months. We had a 60 percent first-day quit rate.

Though increasingly helpless, my father still retained some control over my mother, and he used it zealously. In the afternoon he would insist that she eat the fruit he cut for her, even if she wasn't in the mood. At the dinner table he would insist that she finish the food on her plate, even if she wasn't hungry. She would do so quietly, if grudgingly; she had no energy to waste on fighting with him. Still, she would get beaten down by my father's constant admonishments, out of a kind of devotion that had turned malignant, to eat more, gain weight, exercise, eat fruits, do things the right way, his way. "It is because I love her," he would tell me when I demanded to know why he always felt the need to be on her case. Certainly he did love her, but the knowledge that there was no respite or hope for recovery, that despite all his efforts the course of her disease could not be altered, sapped his spirit and left him angry and embittered.

They had always had different ways of relating to the world. She was cautious and even-tempered; he was often impulsive. She was content, a homebody; he was ambitious and had wanderlust. She was raised in an affluent New Delhi home with servants; he grew up in poverty in rural Kanpur. She was smooth and sociable; he was stubborn and eccentric. In its early years their marriage was a tinderbox. There was unresolved anger, bitterness toward in-laws—almost anything could trigger an inferno of invective and tears. But with time they grew to understand one another. She accepted his idiosyncrasies with a kind of bemused resignation, as if they had been written in the stars, just part of the deal of an arranged marriage, and she resolved to make the most of it. She did not believe in talk or analysis or drama, only in putting your best foot forward and grinding ahead, accepting your circumstances with dignity and grace.

Those traits of my mother persisted even as her physical condition declined. One evening shortly after the move, I was helping her up the stairs to her bedroom. She was walking slowly; after several recent spills, she was terrified of falling again. But even as she struggled, her hands turning white as she gripped the banister, she turned to me and said, "This must be so hard for you."

We wanted our parents to remain in their own home for as long as possible, as they wanted, which meant that my siblings and I were going to have to chip in to help. It was a small price to pay, we thought, for our parents' continuing to live independently. During her frequent visits from Minneapolis, my sister would bathe and dress my mother. I administered her medications and helped with groceries. My brother took care of household issues. Still, my parents' home, like my parents themselves, was in a constant state of disrepair.

That summer of 2014, my siblings and I joined the ranks of the 15 million or so unpaid (and untrained) family caregivers for older adults in this country. A study in 2016 found that the busiest half of this largely invisible workforce spends, on average, nearly thirty hours a week providing care to relatives, many with dementia—an estimated more than $400 billion worth of annual unpaid time. The work takes its toll.* These family caregivers are at increased risk of developing depression as well as physical and career difficulties, including loss of job productivity. Being sick and elderly in this country can be terrifying. Having a sick and elderly loved one is often a full-time job.

"It was the hardest unpaid job I have ever had," wrote a family caregiver in the comments section of an article I wrote in *The New York Times* after my parents' move. "[My father] required 24/7 care so I had to hire an army of caregivers to help, along with trying to manage his medical care, dwindling money, sell his home, move him numerous times, and deal with day-to-day crises. Bless everyone out there that is going through this."

Another person wrote:

"I was both fortunate and unfortunate that my parents were

---

* In a two-year study conducted in 2005, cortisol levels in the morning saliva of fifty-seven caregivers were found to be significantly higher than those of the control group. This was linked to chronic stress.

failing when I was in my 20s and early 30s. Unfortunate because I was young when I lost them and young when I was navigating caring for them while trying to build my own career and life. But fortunate that I had the energy that youth brings to care for them. I do not regret it: they were good parents and when they died, I knew I had done everything I could for them. But it came at a price. I have no spouse, no children, and am now entering my 60s." She added, "As I head towards retirement, I am very much alone in this world."

History can provide some perspective on what is happening. A hundred years ago, most Americans lived in large, multigenerational families, about a third on farms. Today, most Americans live in smaller, detached family units in urban areas. There have been cultural shifts, too. More wives and daughters work outside the home. Children grow up to blaze their own paths. There are benefits to these new freedoms, of course, but also costs. As Americans live longer and with more chronic conditions, they face the prospect of many years of total dependence with fewer relatives around to help care for them. Government support is largely nonexistent.*

After Sharon left, I called a hotline number at the Nassau County

---

* The lack of government support is beginning to change. In 2015, the year after my parents moved to Long Island, Andrew Cuomo, then governor of New York, announced a $67.5 million grant to help ease the burden of the estimated 1 million or so informal caregivers for dementia patients in the state. The money pays for counseling, education, support groups, and a twenty-four-hour hotline. It also subsidizes the hiring of friends and neighbors at $15 an hour so that family members can enjoy occasional respite from the strain of caregiving. They can go and run errands, meet with friends, or even just take a nap. The assistance is available without financial eligibility requirements, so those who don't qualify for Medicaid, which pays for home health aides, have a source of help. Several other states, including North Carolina, North Dakota, Minnesota, and Vermont, have similar programs but on a much smaller scale. However, most states provide no such assistance.

Office for the Aging to find out what resources might be available for my mother. There was nothing unless we could pay. This lack of support applies to most aspects of caregiving for the elderly. For example, of the $200 billion in total annual costs for dementia care, Medicare pays only $11 billion. The shortfall must be covered by families, to the tune of $80,000 per family per year—almost double the outlay for cancer or heart disease.* Long-term care insurance may help with the burden, but most Americans don't own or cannot afford such policies. The U.S. government's approach contrasts sharply with that of other industrialized countries. France and Sweden, for example, spend twice as much on social services for the elderly as they do on their medical care. In the United States, on the other hand, 25 percent of all Medicare dollars are spent on the acute medical needs of 5 percent of patients in their final year of life. Most of that money is spent on hospitalized patients in their last few months.

Medicare does cover some home services, but only after a person has been hospitalized (and then only for a short period, usually a couple of weeks). Patients like my mother who need "custodial" care—assistance with toileting, bathing, or meals—are largely on their own. Hospice care may be available, but only for people who are terminally ill; most elderly Americans do not fit into this group. Therefore, many individuals, like my mother, remain in a sort of limbo: not sick enough to receive government-funded assistance but not well enough to function independently without it. So, unless families can afford to hire private help, most of the burden of eldercare is borne by unpaid caregivers.

---

* In 2018 the average lifetime cost of care for an American with dementia was put at nearly $350,000, with 70 percent being the cost of care at home, including paid help and durable medical equipment, such as wheelchairs. In the absence of government help, families must assume most of this burden.

"No senior citizen/elderly care agency wanted to spend time on the phone with me once it was disclosed there was little money to pay for their services," another caregiver wrote online. "They were not interested in helping my mother who only has Medicare and a small social security check. I understand their response and I understand that these agencies need to make [money] to pay for their staff and facilities and insurance, but I had a rude awakening. The eldercare system in this country is in my opinion heartless and brutal to our frail elderly citizens and their families who have little money."

The comment did not surprise me. It reflects the widespread disenchantment with the profit-driven health care system in this country that I knew all too well from my years in practice. But now my parents were entangled in that system.

Fortunately, my parents had some money saved to pay for my mother's care. My father had a government pension, thanks to his work with the Department of Agriculture, and they both received Social Security benefits. But should my siblings and I try to protect those assets? Should we transfer them to a trust so that our parents could qualify for Medicaid, which covers custodial and nursing home care? More immediately, what about living wills? Health care proxies? Power of attorney? Should we consult an eldercare lawyer? These were just some of the questions we began grappling with in the summer of 2014.

Yet even though our parents' independent living required a steadily increasing financial and emotional commitment, there was no dearth of moments to remind us that it was worth it. One afternoon I called my father from my car to tell him I was going to stop by the house later to fill my mother's pillbox. When we ended the conversation, he forgot to hang up the phone. I heard him turn on the TV, which was playing a popular Hindi film song.

"Will you listen to some music with me?" he asked my mother. She did not reply. "Come on, hold my hand," he said.

"No one has any use for me," I heard my mother say.

"I do," my father said. "The kids do. Here, hold my hand and dance with me."

2

SO, WHEN WILL YOU BRING PIA?

One day during my parents' first winter on Long Island, a few weeks after the visit to Dr. Gordon, my father and I went for a walk. The sun was shining brightly that day, fluorescing off the white drifts to either side of us. The snow had come early that year; it was now melting into a kind of grayish honeycomb along the footpath. Cars in driveways were blanketed in frost. Pellets of road salt crackled under our shoes.

"You tripped here, remember?" I said, pointing to where the sidewalk was jutting up.

My father nodded. He remained a handsome man, with his meticulously trimmed salt-and-pepper mustache, appearing twenty years younger than his age. That afternoon he was wearing a red sweater under his bomber jacket. A green cap with earmuffs covered his head. "I was running," he recalled of the brief stumble that fortunately had not resulted in injury. (He had been walking.) "It was dark."

"You must not go out when it's dark," I admonished. "I've told you before."

"I should go with Pia," he said, laughing. "When will you bring her?"

"I brought her last weekend."

"No," he cried.

"I did."

"Well, you should bring her more often. She's a lovely child."

I told him I would. I didn't have the heart to tell him that his beloved granddaughter rarely wanted to visit anymore.

He stopped to blow his nose with his fingers, leaving a string of snot on the wet snow. "Come on, let's go back," he said. We had walked about a block.

"You don't want to walk some more?"

"No, I'm tired," he said, turning around. Then, as if on cue, the tape rewound. "So, when will you bring Pia?"

As our conversation during that walk revealed, my father's most troubling symptom that winter was short-term memory loss. But, I began to wonder, what exactly is memory? How is it encoded in the brain, and what causes it to deteriorate in dementia?

These weren't just academic questions to me. As a doctor, but also as my father's son, I felt compelled to explore these questions in part by digging into the science of brain degeneration. Understanding my father's condition at a deeper level, I hoped, would help me make sense of what he was going through, and what we as a family might expect in the months and years ahead. At the same time, I believed that confronting his memory loss would help me cope with the emotional and practical dilemmas that arise when someone you love becomes a different sort of person. I would investigate broadly, from deep questions such as what makes us who we are and how to honor my father's wishes for his future self to more specific matters such as the utility of medications and the existence of novel therapies and caregiving strategies. Knowledge, I believed, would give me insight, a deeper sense of the situation, but also empathy (though this didn't always work out as planned). In the coming years, it would be when my father's behavior seemed random, incomprehensible, with no purpose or blueprint, that I was most frustrated as a caregiver. Thus, acquiring knowledge of the science and history of his condition not only illuminated his needs but allowed me to take better care of myself, too.

One of the first accounts of memory loss that I read that winter was the fabled case of a man who lost his ability to form memories. For several years, his story was what I would turn to in order to understand what was going on inside my father's brain and what was in store for him and us.

Henry Molaison (or H.M., as he was known for reasons of privacy in the scientific literature until his death in 2008) was born in 1926 in Mansfield, Connecticut, a small town about ten miles east of Hartford. The only child of an electrician and a homemaker, he had an unremarkable childhood until the age of ten, when he began to suffer from seizures. They started after a bicycle accident (though the accident is not thought to have caused the seizures). In the beginning, the episodes were mild. Molaison would open his mouth and close his eyes, or sometimes scratch his arms or sway like he was daydreaming, until he would wake up, shaking his head and saying, "I've got to come out of this." However, by the time he turned fifteen, the seizures had evolved into more serious episodes involving tongue biting, urinary incontinence, and profound postseizure confusion.

Already quite shy, a science geek and a loner, Molaison became even more socially isolated because of his debilitating condition. He dropped out of high school and lived with his parents (though he eventually went back to earn his diploma at the age of twenty-one). Though he had an above-average IQ, he struggled to hold steady employment. For a time, he repaired electric motors at the Underwood Typewriter plant in Hartford. All the while, and despite treatment

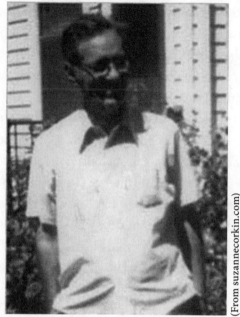

(From suzannecorkin.com)

Henry Molaison

with high doses of antiepileptic drugs, his seizures progressed. By his early twenties, he was having them about ten times a day.

In 1943, when he was seventeen, his family doctor referred him to Dr. William Scoville at Hartford Hospital. A neurosurgeon, Scoville specialized in lobotomies. Over the years he had cut out varying amounts of the temporal lobes of thirty schizophrenic patients to alleviate their psychosis, though with little success. Since seizures sometimes originate in the temporal lobe (though brain-wave studies at the time suggested this was not the case for Molaison), Scoville considered performing a lobotomy on his teenaged patient. However, because Molaison was so young—and studies were inconclusive as to the cause of the seizures—Scoville decided instead to put him on more medication and monitor the response. For ten years he tried to manage his patient's seizures with the highest tolerable doses of the anticonvulsants Dilantin and Mesantoin, the antiepileptic Tri-

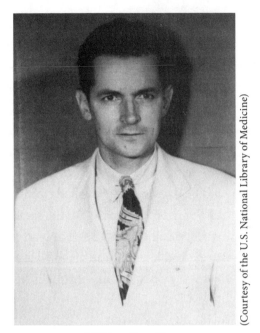

(Courtesy of the U.S. National Library of Medicine)

William Scoville

dione, and the barbiturate phenobarbital, but to no avail. In the end, with nothing else to offer, Scoville proposed the surgery he had originally considered: a lobotomy that would excise several important structures, including the olfactory lobes, which regulate smell; the amygdala, which controls emotions; and the hippocampus, whose function was not properly understood at the time. "This frankly experimental operation was considered justifiable because the patient was totally incapacitated," Scoville later wrote. Exhausted and desperate for relief, Molaison, then twenty-seven years old, and his parents agreed to proceed.

So, on August 25, 1953, several months after Dr. Jonas Salk made the first announcement of his polio vaccine, Scoville drilled two half-dollar-sized holes about five inches apart in Molaison's skull just above the orbits of his eyes and, careful to avoid injuring large blood vessels, suctioned out a small cupful of tissue from each of his medial temporal lobes. The excised tissue included most of the amygdala, the hippocampus, and the anterior temporal cortex on both sides.

Molaison's seizures did abate after the operation (though they persisted in a milder form for the remainder of his life). However, he now had even bigger problems, which manifested almost immediately: he could not remember who his hospital caregivers were, no matter how many times he was introduced to them. He got lost going to the bathroom, no matter how many times he was shown where it was. As with my father, daily events vanished from his mind almost as soon as they had occurred. He would tell the same story over and over, unaware that he had already told it. He read the same magazines, unaware that he had already read them. "He seemed to recall nothing of the day-to-day events of his hospital life," Scoville and a colleague, the neuropsychologist Brenda Milner, wrote in a paper describing the unusual case.

Molaison's *working* memory was fine. Working memory is a form of short-term memory that sifts through our sensations and perceptions and holds on to the ones that are most useful to us in the moment. It is of brief duration—about fifteen to twenty seconds, on average, in a normal adult—thus enabling our brains to temporarily store and manage the information required to perform everyday tasks.* Indeed, Molaison was able to hold on to information for half a minute or so after it was presented (longer, if he actively rehearsed it), so he could carry on a conversation or eat a meal without forgetting

---

* Working memory improves throughout childhood, reaching peak performance in early adulthood. It declines again in old age. A normal working memory can hold between five and nine items—what the psychologist George Miller called "The Magical Number Seven, Plus or Minus Two," the title of his influential paper in *Psychological Review* in 1956—but the information decays unless it is actively rehearsed. For example, when you hear a new phone number, you may remember it for a while—it may eventually be transferred into long-term memory, if it is important—but more often than not the information will be discarded and forgotten if it is not attended to.

what he was doing. But once a task was completed, it got erased like an Etch A Sketch drawing, never to be remembered again. This condition is called *anterograde amnesia.*＊

Surprisingly, most of Molaison's other cognitive functions remained intact. He continued to have above-average intelligence and language skills, and his existing memories were largely spared, too. He could still remember vacations with his parents, jobs he had held as a teenager, going target shooting with his father, and other events from his childhood. Yet, like so many patients living with dementia, he could form no *new* long-term memories. New experiences slipped through his fingers like grains of sand never to be touched again. With no new memories, he lived in a perpetual present, disconnected from his past (or at least the past after his surgery) and his future. It was "like waking from a dream," he said. "Every day is alone in itself."

Milner, who trained at Montreal's McGill University with the famous Canadian psychologist Donald Hebb, and Scoville commenced an in-depth study to investigate the connection between Molaison's brain surgery and his memory deficits. In 1957, in a landmark paper titled "Loss of Recent Memory After Bilateral Hippocampal Lesions," published in the *Journal of Neurology, Neurosurgery and Psychiatry*, they reported their patient's "striking and totally unexpected" amnesia for the first time. Though psychologists and philosophers had

---

＊ In Christopher Nolan's movie *Memento*, Lenny, the main character, who is loosely based on Henry Molaison, has severe anterograde amnesia. He retains long-term memories, such as the fact that his wife has been murdered, but he forgets new people and experiences immediately. So he takes to writing things down. Because he forgets where he puts the slips of paper, he begins to tattoo information on his body. Unable to gauge the veracity of anything anyone tells him, he is vulnerable to manipulation and deception, sadly even by himself. At the end of the film, he discards the scrap of paper telling him who killed his wife so he can continue his never-ending quest to find the killer, which adds purpose and meaning to his life.

long argued that memory functions were widely distributed in the brain, Scoville and Milner's results suggested otherwise. Correlating their observations of Molaison with data on nine psychiatric patients who had received similar operations, the researchers noted that the degree of memory loss was proportional to the volume of medial temporal lobe removed. This suggested to them that a structure in the medial temporal lobe was "critically concerned in the retention of current experience." That structure, they concluded after detailed study, was the seahorse-shaped hippocampus (and the adjacent hippocampal gyrus). Furthermore, because Molaison retained memories of events before his surgery, they deduced that the hippocampus was not the ultimate storage site for long-term memories. That place was in a part of the brain untouched by Scoville's scalpel.

Milner and another neuropsychologist, MIT's Suzanne Corkin, studied Molaison for decades. (Despite this long association, each time Molaison visited them he acted like he was meeting them for the first time.) The researchers learned that their patient's memory deficit was limited to new personal experiences (such as whether he had eaten lunch that day) and new facts about the world (such as the name of the current president). Cognitive psychologists now call such memories *explicit* or *declarative* (because people can talk about them).

However, explicit memory is only one type of long-term memory. There are also implicit memories ("muscle memory") of how we do things. In 1945, in a famous address to the Aristotelian Society in London, the philosopher Gilbert Ryle made a distinction between "knowing that" (a piano is a musical instrument with keys, for example) and "knowing how" (to play a sonata). "Knowing that" is explicit knowledge about a particular thing. "Knowing how," on the other hand, is unconscious, procedural knowledge that cannot necessarily be articulated (and therefore is termed *implicit* or *nondeclarative*). For instance, you may know how to ride a bicycle without being able to describe each separate action required to stay balanced on two moving wheels.

"The advance of knowledge does not consist only in the accumulation of discovered truths," Ryle wrote, "but also and chiefly in the cumulative mastery of methods." In other words, explicit (declarative) and implicit (procedural) memories are distinct. Are they also processed in different parts of the brain?

Indeed, in 1962, Milner discovered that even though her now-famous patient could not form new declarative memories, he was still able to learn new motor skills. In a pivotal study, she trained him to do a complex procedural task: tracing the outline of a five-pointed star while looking at his hand and the star in a mirror. It is a difficult task that anyone would struggle with, and Molaison had a hard time with it at first. However, though he could never explicitly remember having done it before, he got better with practice. "This is strange," he would say. "I thought that would be difficult, but it seems as though I've done it quite well." Thus, despite Molaison's profound amnesia, his procedural memory seemed largely intact.

Other types of implicit memory were undamaged, too. For example, asked first to discuss the meaning of the word "episode," he was more likely, in a word-completion task a few minutes later, to complete the stem "epi" as "episode" rather than, say, "epic" or "epilepsy." This occurred even though he had no conscious memory of the previous conversation. The creation of memories in this way is called *priming* and uses cortical areas that remained intact in Molaison's brain.

Today we know, as Scoville and Milner showed in their landmark paper, that explicit long-term memory is formed by the hippocampus and its associated structures. This anatomical association is important because the hippocampus is often the first structure damaged in Alzheimer's disease, which is why patients like my father often cannot remember recent events, such as what they ate for lunch, though they may retain memories from childhood or early adulthood.

Implicit long-term memory, on the other hand, is served by different brain structures. Procedural memory, for example, relies on the cerebellum and the basal ganglia, which are damaged in Parkinson's disease—though not in Alzheimer's until the later stages. This may be why my mother could remember *when* she bought an article of clothing but not *how* to put it on (and my father vice versa). I learned later that patients with even advanced Alzheimer's disease can often still take part in activities such as walking, dancing, or singing that rely on embodied procedural memory. They may even remember how to play the piano or ride a bike. Knowing-how in such patients persists much longer than knowing-that.

Due to his particular memory deficits, Molaison's life after his operation was difficult. He lost his job at the typewriter plant but eventually found employment at a work center near Hartford, doing simple tasks like packing balloons into small bags (though he could never remember exactly how many he was supposed to pack). He had a hard time making friends because he immediately forgot anyone he met. At home he would forget a family member was dead and appear shocked and sad every time he was reminded of the fact. (He took to carrying around a piece of paper reminding him that his father had died.) With every blink of the eye, his present was seemingly wiped clean, never to resurface again. "How long have you had trouble remembering things?" a researcher asked him in 1992. "I can't tell you," Molaison replied, "because I don't remember."

In his later years, Molaison was able to acquire odd bits of new knowledge, such as recognizing certain personalities, like President Kennedy or Ray Charles, who had become famous after his operation, probably because of repetitive exposure to them in the weekly magazines he loved to read. As he grew older, he retained the gist of childhood memories, but none of the vivid details that gave them life. This suggested, in yet another important insight gleaned from his case, that the hippocampus may be necessary for not only the encoding but also the retrieval and upkeep of personal memories.

An agreeable man, Molaison continued to undergo memory testing for the remainder of his life, never tiring of it because it was always new to him. "It's a funny thing," he once cracked to a scientist at MIT. "You just live and learn. I'm living, and you're learning."

After his death at the age of eighty-two from respiratory failure in a long-term care facility in Connecticut in 2008, his brain was fixed, frozen, and sectioned into more than two thousand slices. Photographs show the overall topography to be relatively normal, save for the five-centimeter voids where his hippocampi and their surrounding structures had been.

The operation weighed heavily on Scoville, the surgeon. He regretted the outcome and, in a 1974 lecture, lamented the surgery as a "tragic mistake." Nevertheless, Scoville's mistake was a gift to neuroscience, providing unparalleled insights into the nature of human memory and how it is lost. It showed that there are multiple memory systems in humans (and presumably other primates), and it confirmed that short-term and long-term memories are distinct, as the eminent psychologist William James had proposed in 1890. It proved that the medial temporal lobe, specifically the hippocampus, is essential for encoding explicit long-term memories, although those memories, once made, reside somewhere else in the brain. Most important, it showed that language and intellect are brain functions distinct from memory. A person without memory can still be intelligent. Despite the destruction of his memory, Molaison retained his above-average intelligence until he developed dementia in his final days.

3

THEN I WILL TAKE A TAXI

My father had been badgering us to help him set up scholarships for underprivileged students at a university on Long Island. Rajiv and I ultimately selected Hofstra, in the town of Hempstead, where I was teaching a first-year course on cardiology at the medical school. Within a few months after my parents arrived, we had created the Dr. Prem and Mrs. Raj Jauhar Endowed Scholarship for disadvantaged students who demonstrate superior academic achievement. The university recommended an unrestricted scholarship, but my father insisted that the award's mission statement specify that "preference will also be given to students who enhance the diversity at the University."

At the farewell luncheon in Fargo a few months before he retired, my father had been recognized for similar scholarships he'd created at North Dakota State for "academically bright but financially stressed" foreign students. In a surprise tribute, the chancellor presented my father with a university plaque and announced that the university's new diversity and equity center would be named in my parents' honor. Afterward, with much of the family in attendance, my father addressed the hundred or so assembled guests. "I know firsthand what it means to be poor, what it means to be hungry, and what it means to be without books," he said to the people sitting before white tablecloths and sipping wine. "This is why I organized these scholarships. My only goal in life now is to help the poor and the needy. If I can help a hungry child or a widow, that will be the best use of my money. My philosophy has always been 'Keep moving toward your goal; it doesn't matter if you reach it. Success is a journey, not a destination.'"

His early life, he recounted that rainy April day, had been a struggle. At age eight, he escaped with his extended family, including six siblings, from what is now Pakistan during the partition of India in 1947. Traveling in oxen-drawn wagons along rutted roads, they somehow evaded the sectarian violence that accompanied partition, spending nights in abandoned train stations among trampled luggage and fresh corpses from the religious massacres. They made it out of the country, but months of squalor in border camps, where cholera and dysentery were rampant, would claim the lives of my father's grandmother and his youngest brother. The family of eight eventually settled in Kanpur, three hundred miles southeast of New Delhi, in a one-bedroom flat without electricity or running water. With no money to buy school supplies, my father did his homework with borrowed books under streetlamps. Each morning he would walk nearly four miles to the academy because the family could not afford to buy him a bicycle. My grandmother had to sell her jewelry to pay the tuition (and bribes) for him to go to college, making him the first in his family to pursue higher education. Twenty-three years after starting college, he immigrated to the United States under the category of "scientists of exceptional ability."

A few months after he created the scholarship at Hofstra, my father was invited to a luncheon the university held to thank him and other benefactors. I postponed a lecture I was scheduled to deliver at the medical school that day so I could accompany him. Of course I was proud of his generosity and dedication to using his savings to further the cause of higher education for minority students. But I was also afraid to let him make the fifteen-minute drive—not to mention attend the two-hour luncheon—by himself.

The wind was gusting when I pulled into my father's driveway late in the morning on the appointed day. He was nattily dressed in a gray three-button suit, one he might once have worn giving plenary talks at international conferences. Just as he got into my car, a curtain of black clouds descended, a few drops on the windshield heralding a deluge. For several minutes we sat in parked silence as sheets of rain skidded across the glass and the heavy sky roared, releasing its tension.

After the brief storm had passed, I backed out of the driveway and eased my car onto the flooded street. "Use both hands," my father instructed as we crashed through puddles on the pitted road. We drove under a graffitied underpass and onto the main thorough-fare. Though he had been in Hicksville for months, I realized we had never driven through the town together. That morning we saw it in all its heterogeneous glory. Hicksville had its share of bustling Indian temples and eateries, but also more than a few ramshackle buildings with cracked facades on abandoned lots. South Asian immigrants were the mainstay of the depressed local economy, bringing in both investment dollars and the entrepreneurial spirit characteristic of the Indian subcontinent's diaspora.

Driving past Patel Brothers market, I couldn't help but remember a time, in the early years after our move to America in 1977, when the roles were reversed—when my parents would pile us into their old Ford Maverick in Lexington, Kentucky, and take us to Kroger or MRS Foodtown on Saturday night to buy groceries. Rajiv and I would race the rusty metal cart up and down the aisles under the white fluo-rescent lights, buzzed on the scent of fresh-roasted chicken—America, the Land of Plenty!—grabbing boxes of frozen pizzas and TV din-ners, tormenting our poor mother. The produce in America was so exotic, so different from the guavas and chikoo fruit sold by the wizened men who pumped their muscled legs on the bicycle-drawn wagons in the lane behind our cement flat in New Delhi. At the supermarket, my parents would occasionally see an Indian family and stop to say hello, so rare was it in those years (at least in the places where we lived) to meet fellow immigrants. Then, more often than not, I would see them at our house for dinner a week later and start calling them "Auntie" and "Uncle."

We had moved to America as beneficiaries of liberalized U.S. immigration policies for scientists and academics. Though I'd largely grown up in the United Kingdom we'd spent the previous year in India, where our apartment in New Delhi was on a dusty dirt road. Farm animals roamed the streets amid the fumes of dung and diesel exhaust. I was only seven years old, but I still remember the austerity, thrown into relief against the relative luxury of our four years in the United Kingdom. I bathed with a bucket and mug. My mother would boil water on a kerosene stove so that I could have a warm bath. We slept on rope beds under mosquito netting. The toilet was a hole in a cement floor. Every few days my mother would send me to a tiny milk shop to fetch freshly drawn buffalo milk. The proprietor, dressed in an unwashed white dhoti and chewing betel leaf, would pour the milk into my tin pail and hock brown spit at crates of Fanta on the mud floor. I would nervously give him the folded bills my mother had sent with me and then run home, my pail swinging wildly, the warm milk sloshing with each panicked stride. Back at the flat, my mother would light the stove to boil the milk to pasteurize it, just as she boiled the water for our baths and for us to drink.

On school days, my father and I would leave home just after dawn, the pungent smell of sewage wafting from open gutters. My fingers would ache as he squeezed them while we crossed the crowded roads, trying to avoid the bullock carts and the roaming white cows. At the crowded bus stop, or sometimes in the park on the way there, he would force-feed me an overripe banana. On the bus I would set my lunch box on the metal seat and look out on the congested streets—at the three-wheelers with their horns blaring, the small Fiat scooters carrying ladies in silk saris sitting sideways—and pray that I would somehow see my father again at the next stop.

It was a trying year for all of us, but perhaps most of all for my father. "I went back because I was patriotic," he once told me. "I wanted to serve my country, serve the Green Revolution." He believed in the principles of that revolution, which made virtual celebrities of plant geneticists and breeders in India in the 1960s. Having grown up in a country of famine, he had devoted his professional life to the genetic modification of crop plants, especially wheat and millet, to make them hardier, more resistant to scab, and equipped to produce more grain to feed India's poor. The work—methodical and meticulous—appealed to his character, his predilection for microscopic detail, even as it gave him an outlet for his social-minded pursuits. He often quoted a king's speech from Jonathan Swift's *Gulliver's Travels*: "Whoever could make two ears of corn, or two blades of grass, to grow upon a spot of ground where only one grew before, would deserve better of mankind, and do more essential service to his country, than the whole race of politicians put together." Those lines could have served as a mission statement for his research endeavors, if not for the Green Revolution itself.

My father would have preferred to stay in India to continue his work producing high-yield grains while furthering the progress of agricultural science on the subcontinent. But shortly before we went back in September 1975, Prime Minister Indira Gandhi declared a state of "national emergency," suspending the constitution, disbanding opposition political parties, and rounding up politicians and academics and throwing them in jail. The resources and national will to promote scientific research disappeared almost overnight. "It is a problem with the country," I remember him telling my tearful mother. "It is not my fault." To advance his scientific ambitions, we were going to have to leave.

The American Embassy in those days was in a spacious and leafy part of New Delhi barricaded with cement blocks and fringed with barbed wire. On the autumn morning we went to apply for immigration visas, a clerk sitting at an old desk with a typewriter and sundry paperwork told my father that there were no more appointments to be handed out that day. "Then we will wait," my father said. Some hours later, a senior embassy official brought him to the back to tell him that because of immigration restrictions, he would be allowed to apply for visas for only two children. "You will have to leave your daughter," she advised. So my father applied for only four visas, figuring he would have more luck appealing later for an exemption for my sister, who had not yet turned three years old. The ploy worked. A sympathetic immigration officer ultimately agreed that my parents could not leave their baby girl behind.

Thus, my father joined the "brain drain" out of India in October 1976, immigrating to the United States under the category of "scientists of exceptional ability." (The rest of the family stayed with relatives in London for three months until my father secured a job.) The process was supposed to take four years, but the approval for him, my mother, my brother, and me (the documents for my sister came later) was granted in six weeks.

As immigrants to America, my parents lived cautiously, aware, as all immigrants are, of what could go wrong, but they had a sense of optimism, too—perhaps the most authentic kind—which led them to leave their homeland for a life in a foreign country without any assurance of success. It still astounds me that my father moved across continents with a wife and three young children and no money, job, or source of income, even as it saddens me that a man who took such bold risks could not properly organize his final move.

The scholarship luncheon was being held in a vast, high-ceilinged auditorium in the Hofstra student center, about eight miles from my father's house. Smiling and well-dressed representatives from the Office for Development greeted us when we arrived. Plates of salad and salmon had already been laid out on white tablecloths, along with baskets of rolls, pitchers of ice water, and bottles of soda. We were seated next to a distinguished-looking older woman wearing expensive jewelry and salon-done blondish hair who had brought along her granddaughter. My father's face brightened when he saw the pretty girl, who could not have been more than ten years old. He pulled out his wallet, removed a dollar bill, and offered it to the child. "Here you go, young lady," he said, reaching out to her with a slight tremor. The girl stiffened and pulled closer to her grandmother. "Not now, Dad," I said softly, putting my arm around him, but he pulled away from me, his hand still extended. The woman smiled and politely accepted the gift. "She is pretty, like her mother," my father said.

"Oh, that's just epigenetics," the woman said, smiling.

We ate lunch—or rather, my father did; I quietly monitored him, impatient for the ceremony to begin. "Eat something," he urged, pushing a salad plate over to me, but I set it aside; I wasn't hungry. "You're crazy," he muttered, chewing a mouthful of goat cheese and spinach. "It's good food."

After he was finished with the first course, my father took it upon himself to introduce me to the other guests at the table. "This is my son," he announced. "He is the director of cardiology. [I was not.] From the beginning, he was on the top." I cringed as people smiled politely.

"Here, Dad," I said, picking up a bottle of Coca-Cola. "Let me pour you something to drink."

I wasn't wholly embarrassed, not really. The expression I must have worn was rather an appeal for understanding. My father, I was trying to convey, was no longer himself, and it was not my fault. My traitorous eye rolls were an attempt to invite pity—for myself, not him—and to make it clear that I did not approve of, and therefore could not be held responsible for, anything he might say or do.

When I look back at my reactions during this time, I realize that they were motivated in large part by fear. Of all his children, I was the closest to my father, perhaps because we were the most alike. We shared the same physical features: dark skin (for Punjabis), lean stature, big hands and feet. We had similar ambitions; we both craved public recognition, for example, and we were both motivated to write books. We shared many of the same character traits, too: commitment and perseverance, but also self-righteousness, melancholy, and a certain insecurity and inflexibility. Like my father, I firmly believed in the importance of genetics and heredity in the determination of human fate. And as a disciple of this philosophy, I could not help but worry that what was happening to him was going to happen to me, too.

Ever since that first visit to Dr. Gordon, I'd been reading about the role of genetics in dementia. Early-onset Alzheimer's, which usually occurs before the age of fifty-five, is primarily a genetic disease, but more typical, late-onset dementia—like my father's—also has hereditary risk factors. The ε4 allele of the apolipoprotein E (APOE) gene, which affects cholesterol transport inside the brain, is found in more than half of patients with late-onset Alzheimer's, with a frequency more than double that in the general population. This gene confers a threefold risk of developing Alzheimer's if one copy is present, and an eightfold risk with two copies. Additional research has found that several other genes, most of them controlling immune-system activity in the brain, are also implicated in the development of Alzheimer's.

However, genetics don't tell the whole story. The genesis of Alzheimer's, I was learning, is extremely complicated: vascular damage, tissue inflammation, and possibly toxins or other injuries that accumulate with age also come into play. Confounding these observations is the fact that people don't start with the same number of brain cells, and brains with more cells have more cognitive reserve. A further complication is that education and social connections may also improve cognitive reserve, as well as the brain's ability to function in the face of cellular damage. So, in the end, perhaps dementia is simply a math problem: how many neurons survive hereditary and environmental insults versus how many succumb.

As the banquet was winding down, the chancellor of the university, a law professor, came up to the podium to make a few remarks. Under an American flag, he spoke about the mission of widening access to higher education and thanked the donors for their generosity. His assistant then called the benefactors up one by one so the chancellor could thank them personally. By the time my father's name was called, my heart was jackhammering. I led him quickly across the auditorium, his fingers tight in my sweaty palm as we navigated through a maze of tables. When he slowed down in front of the podium to acknowledge the applause, I yanked him forward, afraid that he might try to say something.

At the podium, my father and the chancellor shook hands, and my father graciously received an engraved plaque. My hand on his shoulder, I then guided him back to our table, appreciating the grateful nods of staff and other patrons along the way. I sat down with a huge sigh of relief. I had been so worried about how my father would handle the whole affair; fortunately it had passed without any major mishaps.

But then, with his part of the ceremony over, my father decided it was time to leave. It was almost two o'clock, and he wanted to go home to take a nap.

"We'll leave in a few minutes," I whispered. "Just let them finish."

"I am tired, Sandeep," he said loudly as another name was called. "I did not want to come for so long."

"Please, Dad," I said under my breath. "It doesn't look good if we get up now. We'll leave in a few minutes when it's all over."

He thought about this for a moment. By now people were giving us sideways glances. "Then I will take a taxi," he said, making to get up.

I tugged at the sleeve of his jacket. "Please, Dad," I hissed through clenched teeth. "I work here. Just give it a few more minutes." Then, my chest filling with contempt for him, I said, "Where are you going to get a taxi? You don't even know where you are."

He stared at me, perhaps considering what I had just said, or maybe because he felt humiliated. I am not sure. Then he sat down as it dawned on him that his was not a viable plan.

As the ceremony continued, I looked blankly across the room, shaken from having spoken to my father so bluntly (and in public). I noticed a line of Mylar balloons tied to a banister behind the podium, and a short snippet of a memory began to play in my mind. I am seven years old. There is my father, bursting through the front door of our apartment in New Delhi, carrying a helium balloon. Before he can even sit down, I grab the balloon, run outside to the front of our flat, and let it go. It quickly sails up out of my reach as I jump for it in panic. With his long arms outstretched, my father whisks the ribbon out of the air before it floats away and hands it back to me.

Even as the flickering movie played, I heard him say again, "Let's go, Sandeep, I am tired." No remembrance or resentment: the Etch A Sketch had already been wiped clean. Again I tried to negotiate with him—and I did manage to keep him sitting for a few more minutes—but there was no denying him that afternoon. "Come on, Dad," I said, finally standing up, trying to avoid the sympathetic glances of the patrician grandmother sitting next to us. "Let's go home." We left through a side exit.

We did not speak to each other on the way home. When I pulled into his driveway, the sun was shining again. Tiny rain puddles now reflected a bright blue sky.

"Thank you for coming, Sanja," he said, opening the car door. I could tell he knew that I was still upset.

"It was nothing, Dad," I muttered, just wanting to leave.

"No, it was a lot," he said. "I am glad you took me. You are a good son."

I felt a warm flush. Despite the years apart, a kind word from him still made me feel good. "I'll come again tomorrow," I said.

"What time?"

"I don't know. After work. Maybe we can go for a coffee."

He stepped out of the car in his gray suit, looking every bit the academic he had once been. "I am not fond of coffee," he said, before closing the door. "But I am fond of seeing you."

4

WELL, YOUR REPUTATION WILL LIVE ON

"You," your joys and your sorrows, your memories and
your ambitions, your sense of personal identity and free
will, are in fact no more than the behaviour of a vast
assembly of nerve cells and their associated molecules.

—FRANCIS CRICK, *The Astonishing Hypothesis:
The Scientific Search for the Soul*, 1994

Twenty-five years ago, when I was in medical school, I held in my hands the preserved brain of an elderly man who had died of end-stage dementia. It was an unremarkable structure, that beige organ of about three pounds where the man's attention, language, and memory—indeed, most everything that made him uniquely human—once resided. My fingertips caressed the cerebellum, a bush-shaped structure tucked under the cerebral hemispheres that is responsible for balance and coordination. They probed the cerebral cortex, folded into numerous convolutions, called *gyri*, that increase its surface area (and therefore processing power). Because of the chemicals used to preserve it, the organ had the hard and rubbery consistency of cooked liver, not the pudding-like consistency it'd once had inside the man's skull. Tissue slides viewed under a microscope would no doubt have shown the characteristic changes of Alzheimer's disease.

The brain had been cut into centimeter-thick slices stacked together, like a set of coasters. I picked up a sliver glistening with formalin. In cross section, white and gray patterns were visible. Gray matter is made up mainly of neuron bodies, while white matter consists of nerve tracts coated with myelin, a fatty insulator. However, the intricate patterns told me nothing of the wondrous capacities once harbored in them. If you look inside a computer—at the microchips, the wiring—you can deduce nothing of its remarkable functions. Same with the human brain. Most of this man's emotional life (the heart and gut may also play a role in emotional regulation), and certainly all his memory and cognition, had emerged from the sliced and quartered structure lying in a puddle of liquid in the steel pan in front of me.

Human brains are modular. Just as large companies build regional plants to minimize transportation costs, the brain has evolved a collection of specialized units to serve distinct functions such as vision, language, spatial reasoning, and, of course, memory.

There, in a curved ridge of tissue in this man's medial temporal lobe, was a hippocampus, composed of several cell layers folded together like a cinnamon roll. It was withered and atrophic—at least so we were told; I had not seen enough normal ones to be able to tell for myself. As neuroscientists learned from Henry Molaison, the hippocampus and its surrounding structures are responsible for the encoding of long-term memories. Damage to these structures in the early stages of Alzheimer's disease explains the anterograde amnesia—the inability to form new memories—that is a hallmark of the disorder (and that my father was now exhibiting). The predominant signaling chemical in the hippocampus is called acetylcholine, which is why pro-acetylcholine drugs such as Aricept are used to treat the failing memories of Alzheimer's patients (though with only modest effect).

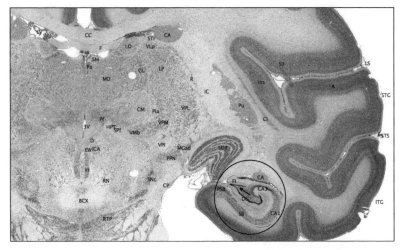

Stained hippocampus with its characteristic cinnamon-roll shape

Hardly a centimeter from the hippocampus was an almond-shaped structure called the amygdala, which regulates emotional responses like fear. The fact that fear and memory structures reside so close to one another is no accident: we must remember what should be feared to ensure our safety and survival. The hippocampus actually goes into a hyperactive state after extreme fear kicks in, rendering certain memories—the topography of a mole on an assailant's cheek, for example—in vivid detail, though other information, such as the layout of the room where an attack took place, may be lost. Such spotty encoding must be kept in mind when we are faced with the often-incomplete recollections of victims of violent crime.

Once memories are made and consolidated, they are no longer

stored in the hippocampus. They become encoded in the neurons of the cerebral cortex, the part of the mammalian brain responsible for higher-order brain functions, such as problem-solving and perception. One of the earliest scientific theories of memory, I learned in my reading, was proposed by Alexander Bain, a Scottish psychologist, who wrote in his 1873 book *Mind and Body* that "for every act of memory, every exercise of bodily aptitude, every habit, recollection, train of ideas, there is a specific grouping, or co-ordination, of sensation and movements, by virtue of specific growths in cell junctions [in the brain]." Bain's insight, it turns out, was essentially correct. Today, memories are believed to depend on the strength of synaptic connections between individual neurons. A network of about a thousand or so neurons and their synapses (the gaps between them)—out of the approximately 100 billion neurons and trillions of synapses that reside in the human cortex—is believed to be sufficient to encode a single episodic memory. When such a network is stimulated by chance or through an effort of recollection, so too are the sensations—visual, auditory, even olfactory—that caused it to assemble in the first place.

Bain's theory was a monumental conceptual leap. For centuries, philosophers had argued that mental phenomena were not reducible to mechanistic events, and that the mind is therefore not embodied in the brain. The most famous proponent of this earlier mind-body dualism was the seventeenth-century philosopher, mathematician, and scientist René Descartes, who attributed to the mind a supernatural status distinct from the physical body. The mind, Descartes believed, was an immaterial entity that could not be reduced to physical flesh. Just as a stone can exist by itself, independent of other entities, Descartes argued, so too can the mind. He wrote in his *Sixth Meditation*: "I have a clear and distinct idea of myself, in so far as I am simply a thinking, non-extended thing [that is, a mind], and on the other hand I have a distinct idea of my body, in so far as it is simply an extended, non-thinking thing. Accordingly, [I am] certain that [my mind] is really distinct from my body and can exist without it."

To Descartes, flesh and soul occupied different domains. Yet in a letter to a clergyman in May 1644, he wrote of "cerebral traces [that] render the brain liable to move the soul in the same way as before, and thus make it remember something; just as the folds in a piece of paper or a napkin make it more apt to be folded that way over again than if it never had been so folded."* Ironically, that insight is the underpinning of the modern scientific theory of memory.

The basic elements of this theory were laid out by the Canadian psychologist Donald Hebb in his landmark monograph *The Organization of Behavior*, published in 1949. Born in Nova Scotia as the oldest child of two doctors, Hebb spent most of his academic career at McGill University in Montreal. He was homeschooled in his early years by his mother, an experience that profoundly affected his later ideas about learning and memory. When he entered public school, he was academically well ahead of his peers and advanced so quickly that he entered high school at the age of twelve. In college he majored in English and philosophy with the intention of becoming a novelist, but when that aspiration did not pan out, he took a job as an elementary school principal while attending evening classes in psychology at McGill, where he eventually earned his doctorate. However, it was his early history of being intensively tutored by his mother that bolstered the insight that propelled his work: that learning and intelligence are not innate but the products of experience.

Hebb, the academic, was puzzled by a surprising anatomical fact: intelligence seems to be largely unaffected by the removal or damage

---

* Descartes was not the first thinker to promulgate this idea. Plato similarly likened memories to etchings on a plate of glass—the deeper the etching, the more permanent the memory.

of even a large amount of brain tissue. "How can it be possible," he wrote, "for a man to have an IQ of 160 or higher (even) after a prefrontal lobe has been removed?"

He was convinced that it was through an increase in the efficiency of the remaining neurons and their connections—a consequence of experience—so that fewer were needed to encode a thought or perception, that the intelligent mind could withstand the excision of brain tissue. Working off ideas proposed by the Spanish neuroscientist Rafael Lorente de Nó, Hebb hypothesized that subjective conscious experiences are encoded in assemblies of neurons that connect together, like a string of Christmas lights. Collective firing strengthens these networks, resulting in a change in the structure and efficacy of their synapses, a process he termed "long-term potentiation."

"The general idea is an old one," he wrote, "that any two cells or systems of cells that are repeatedly active at the same time will tend to become 'associated,' so that activity in one facilitates activity in the other." He did not know how the association occurred, but he hypothesized that it resulted in the lowering of synaptic resistance, the barrier to communication between neurons. This lowered resistance "potentiated" transmission over the same synapses, allowing the networks to fire as independent entities, thus creating discrete and permanent memories. As brain scientists like to say, neurons that wire together, fire together.

In Hebb's theory, the currently accepted model, short-term memory is only a temporary arrangement. If a memory is not attended to, it weakens. To render the memory more permanent, a structural change must take place through repeated firing, a process now known as *consolidation*. In humans, the hippocampus is critical to this process. Though the exact mechanisms are still unknown, it appears that when different areas of the cortex—visual, auditory, olfactory—are activated in a conscious experience, they send signals to the hippocampus, where the various sensations and perceptions are compressed into a cohesive whole.

Then the hippocampus acts as a DJ, replaying the episode over and over again, each time sending signals back to the same areas of the cortex where they originated. The experience is repeatedly, if unconsciously, relived. Once the cortical circuit solidifies, the hippocampus can bow out of the process, and the memory now lives in the cortex. This process often occurs during slumber, which is why sleep is believed to be critical for memory formation.

This process, I came to understand, was the reason why my father, with his deteriorating hippocampus, could still remember events from his childhood, such as the partition of India in 1947, but not what he had just eaten for lunch. The childhood memories were consolidated in cortical networks largely independent of the hippocampus.

The process of consolidation may take days, months, even years, depending on the type and characteristics of a memory. The memory may even change as new information becomes available or old information is reflected upon. For example, I remember that in medical school a neurology lecturer flashed fifteen words in succession on a screen, all having to do with sleep, and asked us, after he was done reading them, to write down as many as we could remember. I wrote down "peace," "yawn," "drowsy," "snore," "slumber," "bed," "rest," and "blanket." After we were done, he asked how many of us had written "bed." Almost everyone raised their hand. He asked how many had written "sleep." Nearly everyone had. But "sleep," he informed us, was not on the list.

"The remembered past is much more fragile, deceptive, and mysterious than we presume," the theologian John Swinton wrote in his 2012 book *Dementia: Living in the Memories of God*. Memory consolidation is a generative process, resulting in modification, manipulation, and reconstruction. Memories may get altered as new information, perceptions, or even emotions change the original experience. They may be reconfigured to conform with our current beliefs. They may end up filled with fictions whose origins are a mystery. When my father eventually (and erroneously) insisted that my mother was sitting on her recliner when she died, he was doing in an exaggerated way what we all do when we unconsciously change the content of our remembrances.

Our memories exist in many places. They live in books, hard drives, smartphones, and other entities external to our minds.* They may even be shared among brains, such as those of a family. Other brains may need to do the remembering when the primary brain fails.

I remember a misty December day, several years before my parents moved to Long Island, when I phoned my father from Central Park after a long run. The wind was whistling that evening. A cold rain had left fallen leaves in heavy sodden piles. My father was telling me about a distant cousin of his who had just died. Like most of my father's relatives, Vikas was someone I had apparently known as a child growing up in India but have no recollection of ever meeting.

"I'm sorry, Dad," I said.

"Yes, well . . ." His voice trailed off.

"How did he die?"

"I don't know, must be something. All my friends are dying. I went to see someone in Delhi, a professor, a class fellow. He was dead, too. Sometimes I think I'd better clear off my desk and get rid of all these papers."

* See Andy Clark, *Supersizing the Mind: Embodiment, Action, and Cognitive Extension* (New York: Oxford University Press, 2008).

The thought of my father's eventual death—that such a terrible experience was in store for me—erased the good feeling from the run.

"Are you afraid of dying?" I asked.

"I am not afraid, but I don't want to die," my father replied without missing a beat. "Too much to do."

"So what do you think comes after?" I asked. "Do you live again or is this it?"

"As far as I am concerned, this is it," he replied grimly. "I don't know if there is anything afterward. No one knows."

The light was shrinking fast. A group of teenagers were sitting on a boulder, giggling and blowing smoke into the haze.

"So what's the point if this is all there is?" I asked.

"Well, your reputation will live on," he answered.

"But you won't know about it, so what's the point?"

The point, he explained, was that there is consolation in knowing that people will remember you, even if you are not around to remember yourself.

As I would soon learn, sometimes we must carry this burden for our loved ones even when they are still around.

5

ONE DAY SHE WILL BE GONE, AND THIS WILL ALL BE LEFT BEHIND

Over the course of the year after his first visit to Dr. Gordon, my father's condition deteriorated, rendering the diagnosis of mild cognitive impairment moot. In 1926, two decades after Alois Alzheimer published his first case report on his eponymous disease, a German psychiatrist named Ernst Grünthal described several characteristic features of Alzheimer's disease, including memory loss, carelessness in work or appearance, dulling of comprehension, and extreme irritability. By the time my parents' one-year anniversary on Long Island rolled around, my father had developed them all.

But he was not alone in his inability to face the true nature of his illness. I too found—or rather tried to find—excuses for his lapses. When he would lock himself out of the house, I would tell my siblings that it could happen to anyone. When he forgot where he put his keys or whether he had taken money out of the bank, I explained that he was exhausted; our mother was sick; anyone would behave erratically in such a situation.

In December 2015, we attended Pia's second-grade Christmas play, *Alice in Wonderland*. My mother could barely make it into the auditorium that night. Getting her down the steep steps, past the squirming little boys and girls in their stiff khakis and baby blue dresses, was a formidable task. My father, however, was in fine form that evening: cracking jokes, teasing children, gallantly picking up dropped programs for the pretty young mothers. Once the show began, he loudly applauded at the end of each scene. But then, sometimes, he applauded *during* a scene if a student onstage would begin to clap as part of the performance. Must be deliberate, I told myself, even as I glanced at him suspiciously in the cramped auditorium. Maybe he knows what he is doing.

However, by the turn of the year, the slipups had become more troubling. In January, he received a traffic ticket after running a red light. In February, he bumped his old Audi into a parked car in the Trader Joe's lot. At first, he vehemently denied he had even gotten into an accident; he relented only after I presented him with the police report showing the broken taillights on the other car. My siblings wanted to take away his keys, but I resisted. Anyone can make a mistake, I told them. It was only right to give him another chance.

But the missteps soon became impossible to excuse. At the Hindu temple, he picked arguments with other worshippers about what he saw as Indian venality. Though my father was an avowed supporter of his homeland, his patriotism had always been leavened with a certain disdain for India's continuing fecklessness and third-world corruption. Unfortunately, these opinions did not sit well with the temple's patrons. He was eventually banned from attending prayers.

His management of his money grew more reckless, too. He would take out large sums of cash from the bank—$700 one day, $2,100 a couple of days later—and leave them sitting around the house. My brother and I begged him to stop—my mother's cast of caregivers was coming and going—but he would not (or could not). We would surreptitiously pocket the cash and deposit it back into his account (and he would not even notice). Still, money and jewelry went missing. Bills were going unpaid, too. One from Banana Republic was already under arrears at a collection agency when Rajiv just happened to find it in a pile of papers on the dining table; they had apparently been trying to contact my father since the previous May. When my brother called to pay the bill, the person on the line put him on hold for twenty minutes, then said she could not speak with him, let alone accept his money, unless he showed power of attorney. "I said I just want to pay the bill, but they won't allow even that," Rajiv texted Suneeta and me. "Lmfao. I am laughing but I am so frustrated."

However, in the end it was a phone call from my father that put a stop to my rationalizations. It happened one afternoon late in the fall of 2015 while I was rounding at the hospital. "I wanted to ask you, Sandeep," my father said offhandedly, "and let me know if you disagree, but should we put your mom in a nursing home?" He said it like he was asking what we should have for dinner, not deciding the fate of his beloved partner of more than fifty years.

"Dad," I said, trying to remain calm, though I was in shock, "where's Mom?"

"Oh, she is right here with me." I heard him turn to her. "I am talking to Sandeep," he said, "about whether we should put you in a nursing home."

My mother began to cry, a piercing, horrible wail.

"I am not saying we should do it, Raj," my father said to her, quickly backtracking. "I am saying we should consider it. It is up to you, too. But they will take good care of you. And, of course, we will visit every day."

That phone call—the matter-of-factness of it, the egregious and oblivious cruelty—finally brought home to me that my father's disease had entered a more advanced stage. For more than a year I had disbelieved what was apparent to the rest of the family. I had offered rationalizations out of fear of what was in store for him (and, perhaps, for me, too). No more. If anything, I now found myself gripped by the opposite (and perhaps even more damaging) conviction: that my father was no longer capable of a normal thought.

Of course I would still acknowledge his remarks, but I rarely responded to or valued what he said—and then only if the remarks had the sheen of normalcy, like his comments on the buffoonery of a certain Republican candidate for president in 2016. If they were strange or idiosyncratic, they—meaning he—would be ignored. He would tell me old family stories, but I would find them unfunny or irrelevant and chide him or hurry him along. No doubt I made him feel worse, lonelier than he already was—not on purpose, of course, but it hardly mattered. Once he was labeled as having a brain disease—a label corroborated by my unforgiving interpretations of his conversation—he became to me a minor character in our family, a miniaturized version of his former self, isolated and confined to ever-shrinking boundaries, as I stared sadly at him from outside the cage.

A similar thing happened with my mother. Once she started hallucinating—a consequence of her Parkinson's (or perhaps the drugs she was taking to treat it)—my siblings and I were inclined to interpret almost all her actions and feelings through the prism of her disease. The social psychologist Tom Kitwood has termed such behavior "malignant social psychology." It is a form of depersonalization. Even my mother's being sad or withdrawn because she could no longer walk properly or because my father was continually fighting with her aides was construed by us (and by her doctors) as evidence of failing neurological processes, not as a reasonable human response to difficult and frustrating circumstances. During those years I was writing a book about the heart in which a central theme was the detrimental effects of psychosocial stress on human health. Yet when it came to my parents, my thinking regressed to a model of disease in which their conditions were purely consequences of cellular pathology. Our parents were constrained and marginalized not just by their diseases but also by our response to them.

I remember a winter evening in late 2015 when my father urgently called me over to the house. My mother was sitting at the dining table, her eyes swollen from crying. Evidently she had accused Sujatha, her new aide—the third one in the past month—of misplacing some blankets. "I keep telling her, there is no blanket, no blanket, but she won't listen," my father shouted in frustration. "I told her, 'If you keep accusing Sujatha, she is going to leave!'"

I pulled up a chair and sat down next to my mother. "Mom, there are no blankets," I said firmly. "Sujatha did not take them, but even if she did, that's okay. They were cheap blankets anyway."

"They may be cheap to you but they are not to me," my mother fired back.

To pacify her, I ran upstairs and poked around in her closet. There were piles of silk suits, a back massager I had given her, still in the box, and some devotional relics. No blankets. "I looked everywhere but I couldn't find them," I informed my mother when I came back downstairs, but she insisted on going up to look for herself. She climbed the steps with more alacrity than usual, holding the banister with her left hand because the right one still hurt from a fall. In the master bedroom I pulled down a bundle from a shelf in the closet and unzipped the plastic bag. "No, those are comforters," my mother said. They were not what she was looking for.

Rummaging through the guest-room closet, I found another pile covered with a bedsheet. I unwrapped it, and there, stacked together in bright colors, were the woolen blankets she had been looking for. "Aha," my mother cried triumphantly as I stood by sheepishly, not knowing what to say. She took a few quick steps out of the room. "Now let's go downstairs and tell your father so he doesn't call me a liar."

That night, as snow fell lightly, my father and I sat quietly at the dining table after my mother went to sleep. He had never been one to lose hope, but even he could tell that my mother was entering the downward spiral of the terminally ill, in which competing problems grow in significance, where the solution to one problem causes another. "I feel sorry for your mother," he said, gazing at the muted newscast on the television. "She is so possessive of her things, and I think, One day she will be gone, and this will all be left behind."

Two weeks after Pia's Christmas play, we celebrated my forty-seventh birthday at my house. At the party, my father and I had a minor brouhaha. He asked my guests for their email addresses so he could correspond with them but then panicked after losing the scraps of paper on which the addresses had been written. When I told him that I would email the addresses to him later, he lost his temper and claimed that I would forget. Then I lost *my* temper, telling him it was pointless to ask for things to be written down when he could not remember where he put them. It was a small squabble on an otherwise festive occasion. By the time we cut the cake and my family and guests belted out "Happy Birthday," all was forgotten.

But a couple of days later, my father phoned me on my way to work, insisting that I come over right away. "Can it wait, Dad?" I said as I sped down a slushy Long Island Expressway. "I am on my way to the hospital."

"This is your job, too," he snapped. "I did it for my mother."

Reluctantly I pulled off the freeway and onto the exit ramp, quickly made two lefts, and got back on going east. I checked my watch. My first clinic patient would be arriving in thirty minutes.

"So now we're supposed to drop everything and go over on a

whim?" I groused on the phone to my brother as I weaved through heavy traffic. "Why? So he can tell me he wants to donate his organs again?"

"I dread the phone calls, too, bro," Rajiv replied sympathetically. "Not Mom so much, but it's a package deal."

He and my father had always had a fractious relationship. Being the eldest son in a traditional Indian family hadn't been easy. As much as Rajiv relished the perks, he had resented the responsibilities: to marry someone my parents would approve of, choose a career they could be proud of, serve as a role model for his younger siblings, and always carry the burden of my father's deep faith in him. When Rajiv was fourteen, he was the one chosen to type and proofread my father's first book, *Cytogenetics and Breeding of Pearl Millet and Related Species*, and he was the only child to receive an acknowledgment. He was the one tapped to stay up all night with my father developing micrographs in the laboratory darkroom. I can still remember the sour smell of photo developer wafting over him when he drifted sleepily into our bedroom before sunrise on Saturday mornings.

My father favored my brother because Rajiv did things the right way—the way my father, with his perfectionist tendencies, wanted them done. And though Rajiv usually grumbled and moaned, in the end he always did what was expected of him—out of guilt, perhaps, or a sense of duty, or maybe because of that primal fear of losing a parent's esteem.

As spray from a haul truck splattered on my windshield, I said, "Maybe we don't love our parents the way we should, or the way other kids do," indulging a sudden feeling of regret.

"I feel no guilt," Rajiv replied flatly. "I am at peace with what I do for them."

"But you are doing it because you have to, not because you want to."

"Some do it out of love," he said. "Others out of duty. I do it out of duty."

Whatever our motivations, this was not the way our parents' old age was supposed to have turned out: with them ailing and living alone while their sons squeezed in short visits between their jobs and other responsibilities. As children we had made promises to care for them—promises that, in truth, had not been kept. We had our reasons, of course: work, families, competing priorities. But in the end the renunciation was a choice like any other in our lives, a consequence of dwindling time, growing responsibilities, and perhaps insufficient inclination, too. In physics, the triple point of a substance, such as water, is that temperature and pressure where the three phases of solid, liquid, and gas coexist. This was the point at which my brother and I found ourselves with our family roles: parents, spouses, and now caregivers—each role in an uneasy and unstable equilibrium with the others.

Speeding down the expressway, it was impossible not to wonder whether my parents would have been better off in India in their old age, at least in the India they had left behind, where relatives were around—a brother around the corner, a cousin down the block—and ready to help when the need arose. "In India we are used to extended families," Vini, my brother-in-law, had told me at my father's retirement party two summers earlier when we discussed my parents' move to Long Island. Life in America, Vini often said, was focused on individual goals at the expense of collective responsibility. That culture had served us well—perhaps even served our parents, too, in their prime—but now that they were sick and needed help, it was woefully deficient. Of course, India had changed since we left. Women now often worked outside the home. Care for elders was increasingly being outsourced to a private, paid workforce, if not to the nursing homes sprouting up in major cities across the country. Still, multigenerational families remained the norm. The prevailing culture continued to be one in which eldercare was given priority, or at least not so easily sacrificed in the service of personal goals.

"You keep pushing for them to stay in the house, but it isn't feasible anymore," my brother said as I took the exit into Hicksville. "I had to go over there again yesterday because he locked himself out of the house."

"That wasn't his fault," I said, coming to my father's defense out of habit. "The front door was locked. He exited through the garage."

"Sandeep," my brother cried, "do you really believe that he can still take care of himself? He can't even work the TV! When was the last time he sent you an email? I don't think he knows how to anymore. You keep talking about letting him drive, but he is going to hurt somebody. You have to get over this concept of independence. Mom and Dad need to move to a different situation. Suneeta and I are on the same page. You are not."

When I arrived at the house, the front door was open. My father, still in his pajamas, was pacing back and forth in the living room like he was rehearsing a speech. The house was beginning to look like a junkyard. Old papers he had been trying to sort through were piled up on the dining table. On the walls were random mementos of old travels: a Tibetan plate, a Swiss clock, all reproductions, distant memories.

My father stopped short when he saw me. "Sit down," he said, pointing to the dining table.

"Dad, I don't have much—"

"Sit down," he cried.

On the table lay my father's laptop and a copy of James Watson's *The Double Helix* that I had presented to him the previous weekend—on my own birthday, no less. He had written the words "I received this precious gift from Sandeep!" on the cover, but otherwise the book appeared untouched.

I sat down on a high-backed chair still covered, more than a year later, with plastic wrap. "So, what is it, Dad?"

He took a moment to compose his thoughts. "You are who you are primarily because of me," he started off. He paused to let the words sink in. "Not entirely, but primarily. I was the one who made you stick with medical school."

However strange it was to hear, there was some truth to this assertion. While I was in medical school, my father had always provided a patient ear and unflagging encouragement whenever my motivation had faltered. "Why are you telling me this?" I said impatiently.

"At your birthday, you only talked about your mom. You hardly said a few words about me. It was embarrassing."

I thought back to my toast, surprised that he even remembered. "So what if I said something about Mom. Don't you think she deserves some credit after all these years?"

"Then you dedicated your book to her, not to me," he said, picking up his copy of my second book, *Doctored*, from the table. "Mention both of us!"

"I dedicated my first book to you."

"You did not."

"I did! You just forgot."

Ignoring me, he took out some letters he had inserted in the pages of my book. "Every letter in this house has Rajiv's name on it," he said, holding up an envelope, his hand trembling.

To avoid collection notices, my brother had transferred all the bills into his name. "You will have to talk to Rajiv about that," I said.

"What for, talk to Rajiv?" my father said, suddenly infuriated. "This is my house!"

"It is your house," I said evenly.

"Then why is Rajiv's name on everything?" He grabbed his checkbook, which had been tucked away in the covers of the book, and tore out a check he had written. "Here is the money for this house," he said bitterly. "From the sale of the house in Fargo. Give it to Rajiv."

He looked smaller, more fragile, than I had ever seen him. "It doesn't matter, Dad," I said, trying to soften my tone. "We are a family."

He opened his laptop, saying he wanted to show me something. I glanced at the clock on the wall. My first patient was surely checking in by now. I waited as he stared at the login page.

"You seem tired," I said.

"I am always tired," he responded.

"Well, you seem more tired than usual. What's wrong? How's Mom?"

He paused for a moment. "She's . . . the same. Last night she said there are people sleeping on the carpet. I said, 'No, Raj, there are not.'"

I tried to think of something to say. I admired how he had supported my mother through her illness, even if I recognized how often, like the rest of the family, he had fallen short. "I am proud of . . ." I stopped. The words sounded empty.

"No, I love your mother," he said quickly. "It is the least I can do. You know how much she sacrificed for us. She used to go and teach in the school in India. She took two buses in the hot sun. She stood by my side when I had no job."

I listened. At that moment my father's mind seemed completely clear.

"We had a good life," he went on. "I got all the awards, the gold medals, the center named after me. She had a good life, too. But we are at the end of our days. Now sometimes I think it is best that we should die."

I shot up out of my chair. "What are you saying, Dad?"

He looked through me, as though focused on something thousands of miles away. "I used to be so productive," he said. "Lectures, PowerPoints, emails. Now . . ." His voice trailed off.

"There is still a lot you can do, Dad," I said encouragingly. "We can go to Cold Spring Harbor like we talked about. Maybe you can teach a summer class there"—I knew this was no longer possible— "or, I don't know, volunteer your time in some other way."

My mother called out to him from the bedroom. She had to go to the bathroom again. Raising his voice, he said he was coming. He turned to me. "I don't think you guys will even miss me. You have your own families now."

"Of course we will miss you," I cried. "We have memories!"

"Oh, maybe two or three days, a week, but you will forget. But your mom will miss me. We spent our life together. I may get angry with her, but she is very precious to me. She was always by my side."

My cellphone buzzed. "I know, Dad," I said, desperate to go.

"You don't know," he cried. "She used to teach in the secondary school. She took two buses in the hot sun. Did I ever tell you that?"

He was standing on the stoop when I got into my car. He waved uncertainly as I backed out of the driveway. I felt a vague longing to stay with him, but I had to go; my patients were waiting to see me.

Then, possessed by a feeling I had not had in years, I opened the car door, ran up the steps, and hugged him. The faint smell of Old Spice on his cotton shirt transported me back to a different time, when he was a different man and I regarded him with awe and fear. Seeing him now, still in his night clothes in the middle of the morning—a man who had once taken pride in his work, in always maintaining control of himself (and others)—was heartbreaking. He had always reminded me of the father in Vittorio De Sica's *The Bicycle Thief*: loving, detached, protective, but somewhat pathetic, too. At that moment I felt like the boy at the end of that film, looking wistfully at his fallen father whom he had once beheld with reverence and respect.

"Thanks, Bubboo," he said as I hugged him. I rubbed his stubbled cheek and kissed him. He patted me on the head and offered a half smile. "There is no replacement for parents," he said, as if the entire episode that morning had been another of the lessons that he had been trying to teach me my entire life. "Remember my mother? She died in my arms."

Eyes welling with tears, I turned and walked back to my car. I did not have it in me to tell him that she did not.

6

IT SEEMS WE ARE DEALING HERE
WITH A SPECIAL ILLNESS

Some of my reading involved tracing the history of how people have viewed aging and mental decline over the millennia. For most of human history, conditions like my father's were believed to be a normal part of aging. Even as far back as ancient Egypt, people thought that old age went hand in hand with memory loss—even if that disorder was thought to originate in the heart. For example, an Egyptian text from the twenty-fourth century B.C. describes an elderly court official whose "heart is exhausted and fails to remember yesterday" who spends "every night becoming more childish."

The Greeks, too, recognized that the mind often decays as the body ages. Plato and Aristotle both wrote in the fourth century B.C. about age-related mental decline—the result, Aristotle believed, of an accumulation of cold black bile that rendered old people useless for high posts "because there is not much left of the acumen of the mind which helped them in their youth." This jaundiced view of old age persisted even as civilization progressed. In the second century A.D., the Roman philosopher and surgeon Galen wrote that "old age is not natural in the same way that feeding and growing are." He likened the aging process to "an inevitable infection of the body" and attributed age-related memory loss to "chilling humors" in the brain. He was wrong, of course, even if his insight that physical changes in the brain can influence the mind was a revolutionary leap.

The first-century B.C. Roman statesman Cicero was one of the first of the ancient philosophers to recognize that old age did not necessarily lead to mental decline. "Senile idiocy," he wrote in his treatise *On the Art of Growing Old*, "is a characteristic, not of all old men, but only those who are weak in will." Cicero believed that an active mental life could postpone or even prevent the decay of the mind, which, he maintained, was like a lamp that grows dim unless it is supplied with oil. "It is our duty to resist old age, to compensate for its defects by a watchful care; to fight against it as we would fight against disease," he wrote, adding that "our physical bodies grow heavy with the weariness of exertion, but our minds are rendered lighter and keener by their constant exercise." In his prescient words we can discern the germ of the idea, now widely accepted, that activities that stimulate the brain can slow cognitive decline. Cicero's musings, however, had little influence on thinking about the matter.

In the Middle Ages and the early modern period, dementia does not seem to have inspired much interest or concern, in part because much deadlier epidemics such as the bubonic plague were ravaging humankind. Still, madness and senility were common features of everyday life, finding expression in art and literature. King Lear, for example, appears to suffer from a kind of dementia marked by poor reasoning, paranoia, disorientation, and psychosis ("Who is it that can tell me who I am?"). Another Shakespearean character, "melancholy Jaques" in *As You Like It*, details a morbid end to the human life cycle:

> Last scene of all,
> That ends this strange eventful history,
> Is second childishness and mere oblivion;
> Sans teeth, sans eyes, sans taste, sans everything.

Chaucer, Boswell, and Swift all wrote of the feebleness of the mind in old age. In Swift's *Gulliver's Travels*, for example, the immortal Struldbruggs develop a horrible, age-related dementing disease, becoming "opinionative, peevish, covetous, morose, vain, talkative, but incapable of friendship, and dead to all natural affection." In a clear nod to hippocampal degeneration, Swift wrote that "they have no remembrance of anything but what they learned and observed in their youth and middle-age, and even that is very imperfect." The Struldbruggs symbolize the horrors of prolonged aging, serving as a warning to those who seek longevity at any cost.

Ironically, Swift himself experienced cognitive decline about a decade after his novel was published. He began to wander, developed memory and language difficulties, and became disoriented, clinical signs that were almost certainly the result of Alzheimer's disease. Writing at the age of seventy to a friend, he reported, "I have entirely lost my memory, incapable of conversation by a cruel deafness, which has lasted almost a year, and I despair of any cure." His biographer, William Lecky, wrote in 1861 that "it was not madness . . . (but) absolute idiocy that ensued." Eventually, guardians were appointed to take control of Swift's affairs. By then, "every spark of intelligence had disappeared," Lecky noted. "It was not till he had continued in this state for two years that he exchanged the sleep of idiocy for the sleep of death."

Popular literature notwithstanding, dementia did not inspire much inquiry in the prescientific era in Europe. The forces that controlled the human mind were thought to be mystical and outside the domain of reason. In those years, the Church was the dominant force for promoting knowledge, and questioning religious doctrine through empiric observation was often seen as heresy, which was punishable by death.

However, this deference to dogma began to lift in the seventeenth century as dementia increasingly came to be viewed as a neuropsychiatric condition that could be understood through rational investigation. For example, anatomists began to probe the brain for clues that could explain mental disorders. Some found that the brains of demented individuals were harder and drier than normal brains, or "pressed by an excess of humidity or cold," as the Swiss anatomist Théophile Bonet put it—though a more celebrated anatomist, the Italian Giovanni Morgagni, later rebutted these observations, writing, "I do not lay so much stress upon [brain] hardness. I would have you know that in some persons whose minds had not been disordered, I did not find the cerebrum less hard." Despite such misunderstandings, the focus on the brain as the source of mental disorder was a remarkable advance because the heart had been considered the repository of emotions and mental life for most of prior history.

By the middle of the nineteenth century, a scientific approach to mental disease was taking hold. Physicians found, as countless doctors have since observed, that the brains of patients who died of dementing diseases were often atrophied and lighter than normal. In his 1860 textbook *Traité des maladies mentales*, Bénédict Morel, a French psychiatrist, characterized loss of brain weight as "an expression of decadence in the human species." Four years later, the British physician Samuel Wilks wrote a description of a shrunken brain lying inside a skull for which it had become too small. "Instead of the sulci meeting," he noted, "they are widely separated and their intervals filled with serum." Brain atrophy soon came to be understood as a defining feature of dementia. Indeed, the fact that the autopsied brains of elderly individuals did not always exhibit atrophy helped to overturn the prevailing belief that dementia was an inevitable consequence of aging.

Also in the nineteenth century, mental disease began to be recognized as a medical condition in need of treatment. The French doctor Philippe Pinel, one of the founders of modern psychiatry, focused on

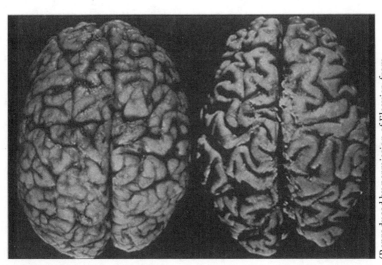

(Reproduced by permission of Elsevier; from N. C. Berchtold and C. W. Cotman, *Neurobiology of Aging* 19 [1998]: 173–189)

Normal (left) and atrophied brains. Brain atrophy was first recognized in the mid-nineteenth century as a feature of senile dementia.

the role of heredity and physiology, rather than moral and religious failings, in the development of insanity. In *A Treatise on Insanity*, published in 1806, he condemned a system that routinely "abandoned the patient to his melancholy fate, as an untamable being, to be immured in solitary durance, loaded with chains, or otherwise treated with extreme severity." At the time, patients suffering from dementia were often locked up with "idiots, epileptics, [and] paralytics," or with prostitutes and other "perverts," and tortured with cold showers and whippings. Pinel's work led to more humane treatment of these patients.

Meanwhile, a classification system for dementia was being created. In France, the psychiatrist Jean-Étienne Dominique Esquirol, Pinel's student, differentiated age-related (or "senile") dementia from other acquired dementias, such as dementia associated with syphilis, which was believed to account for nearly one in ten cases of dementia at the time. Senile dementia, he wrote, "commences with feebleness of memory, particularly recent memory." He added: "Attention becomes impossible; the will is uncertain; the movements are slow." Dementia in that era was commonly referred to as imbecility, foolishness, or idiocy, but Esquirol rightly noted a fundamental difference between dementia and "congenital idiocy," the period term for intellectual disability. "A man in a state of dementia is deprived of advantages which he formerly enjoyed," he wrote. "The idiot, on the contrary, has always been in a state of want and misery."

By the end of the nineteenth century, age-related dementia was believed to be a consequence of reduced blood flow through hardened blood vessels that led to strokes. Neuropathologists commonly described cases of "vascular dementia" in elderly patients whose blood vessels were filled with fatty deposits. However, vascular disease did not explain all cases of dementia, particularly those arising in patients at a relatively young age. Notably, it did not explain what was ailing a fifty-year-old German woman named Auguste Deter, who in 1901 was admitted to Frankfurt's Municipal Asylum for Epileptics and Lunatics, where she was treated by a brilliant psychiatrist named Alois Alzheimer.

Deter was happily married and raising a daughter when she began her descent into madness. In the beginning she had paranoid delusions that her husband of twenty-eight years, Carl, a railway clerk, was having affairs, but her condition soon progressed to amnesia and profound disorientation. She greeted friends as if they were first-time acquaintances. She forgot daily events as soon as they had occurred. Within several months, she was unable to care for herself, prompting her husband to admit her to Frankfurt's "Castle of the Insane," as it was called. "I have lost myself," she told her doctors.

"In the institution, her behavior showed all the signs of complete helplessness," Alzheimer wrote. "She is completely disoriented in time and space. Sometimes she says that she does not understand anything and that everything is strange to her. Sometimes she greets the attending physician like company and asks to be excused for not having completed the household chores. Sometimes she protests loudly that he intends to cut her, or she rebukes him vehemently with expressions which imply that she suspects him of dishonorable intentions."

Though her gait and reflexes were normal, "her memory is seriously impaired," Alzheimer wrote. "If objects are shown to her, she names them correctly, but almost immediately afterward, she has forgotten everything." Her language skills had broken down, too. "When reading a test, she skips from line to line or reads by spelling the words individually, or by making them meaningless through her pronunciation. In writing, she repeats separate syllables many times, omits others, and quickly breaks down completely. In speaking, she uses gap-fills and a few paraphrased expressions ('milk-pourer' instead of cup). Sometimes it is obvious that she cannot go on."

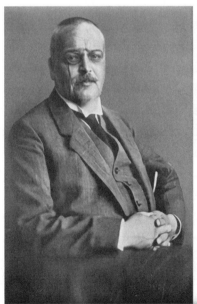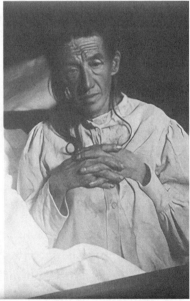

Alois Alzheimer and his most famous patient, Auguste Deter

At the time, Alzheimer was working as a clinical psychiatrist. However, his true passion was neuropathology. As a college student in Berlin, he had become fascinated by the microscopic study of cells. When he returned to Lower Franconia in Bavaria, where he was born, to study medicine at the University of Würzburg, he learned cell staining techniques. After graduating magna cum laude in 1887—his doctoral thesis was on the wax-producing glands of the ear—he was hired at the Municipal Asylum in Frankfurt, where he met Franz Nissl, a neuroanatomist who had invented a special cell stain, the eponymous Nissl stain, still in use today.

The two men became friends, working with patients during the day and spending evenings together at the microscope. Noting his junior colleague's interest in histology—the study of the microscopic structure of tissues—Nissl encouraged Alzheimer to pursue research alongside his clinical work. However, it was only after Alzheimer's wife, Cecilie, the daughter of a wealthy banker, died shortly after giving birth to their third child, thus bequeathing him a large sum of money and making him financially independent, that he took Nissl's advice and devoted himself to laboratory research. By the time his patient Deter died in 1906, Alzheimer had moved to the Royal Psychiatric Hospital in Munich, where he had taken a position as a neuropathologist in the laboratory of Emil Kraepelin, one of Europe's leading psychiatrists. Nonetheless, before leaving Frankfurt he had requested that Deter's medical records and brain be sent to him for study after her death. They arrived in the spring of 1906.

In examining Deter's brain, Alzheimer first noticed significant atrophy. The organ was light in weight and the cerebral cortex thinner than normal for her age. Using newly developed staining techniques, he examined thin slices of the brain tissue under a microscope. He found two puzzling abnormalities. First, "scattered through the entire cortex, especially in the upper layers, [were multiple, tiny] foci that were caused by the deposition of a peculiar substance."

These accumulations are now known as *senile plaques* (Alzheimer called them "buildup products"), and the peculiar substance within them—a brain protein that has undergone structural changes, becoming "sticky" and forming microscopic collections—is called beta-amyloid. Though pathologists had known about amyloid since at least the middle of the nineteenth century (accumulations of different types of it had been observed in many aging organs, including the kidney, heart, and liver), it was not until 1927 that it was identified, with polarized light, as the primary constituent of brain plaques.

The other abnormality that Alzheimer observed, using a special silver stain, was tangles of previously undescribed fibers inside brain cells. "In the interior of a cell that otherwise appeared normal, one or several fibrils stood out due to their extraordinary thickness and impregnability," Alzheimer wrote. These fibrils, electron microscopy later showed, start off as normal structures for transporting nutrients inside neurons but become abnormal when a protein called "tau"

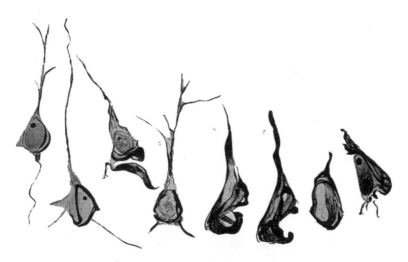

Neurofibrillary tangles and disintegrating neurons
(as drawn by Alzheimer and his colleagues)

misfolds, twisting the fibers into helical shapes, thus interfering with their function.

The fibrils "merged into dense bundles and gradually reached the surface of the cell," Alzheimer wrote. "Finally, the nucleus and the cell itself disintegrate and only a tangle of fibrils indicates the place where a neuron was previously located." Most people over the age of fifty have some such tangles in their brains. It is probably a phenomenon of aging and will not cause dementia in a normal lifespan. However, tangles in the presence of amyloid plaques are much denser and more destructive. And so it was with Auguste Deter's brain. It had disintegrated, its cell bodies flaring into comet-like shapes that bulged with abnormal protein collections. Up to a third of the neurons in her cerebral cortex were affected.

Alzheimer's observations intrigued Emil Kraepelin, his mentor and the most famous psychiatrist in Europe at the time. Kraepelin had long set out to prove that mental disorders originate in brain pathology, and Alzheimer's results resonated with this core belief. He encouraged his protégé to present his findings to the wider scientific community, which Alzheimer first did on November 3, 1906, at a conference of German psychiatrists in Tübingen. However, his lecture, attended by some one hundred people, provoked little interest. (The subsequent lecture on compulsive masturbation seemed to hold more appeal.)

A few months later, Alzheimer published a paper in which he laid claim to a "distinctive disease process" in the brain. "Considering everything, it seems we are dealing here with a special illness," he wrote. However, that paper also garnered little attention.

Nevertheless, Kraepelin was convinced that Alzheimer was onto something important, and so in 1910, in the eighth edition of his influential textbook *Psychiatrie*, he described Auguste Deter's case along with his mentee's findings and dubbed the condition "Alzheimer's disease." He summarized many of the basic features of the disease, including "the decrease in receptivity, decrease of mental resilience, restriction of sentimental relationships, slackening of energy, [and] the development of obstinate unmanageability."

"Patients' emotional life is gradually devastated," Kraepelin wrote. "Their awareness either of suffering or of enjoying life decreases considerably." In most cases, he remarked, "Perceptual and memory impairments appear as the most characteristic symptoms." He noted that "events of their childhood are recalled in their mind with surprising vividness," even as "the memory of recent events starts to reveal numerous and incomprehensible gaps." Kraepelin conceded that the clinical significance of Alzheimer's disease was still unclear. However, because of Kraepelin's outsize reputation, the name stuck, and by the following year it was being used in the United States and Europe to diagnose patients with mental deficits.

Still, progress in understanding the mechanisms of dementia stagnated for several decades. The slow headway was due in part to the fact that Deter had been so young when she became afflicted. Though her symptoms were similar to those seen in elderly patients, a fundamental question remained unanswered: Was "Alzheimer's disease," a term used for relatively young dementia patients like Auguste Deter, the same as the more common dementia observed in elderly adults?

Neither Alzheimer nor Kraepelin believed the two diseases were the same, and they were not alone. Many pathologists maintained that the plaques, tangles, and neuronal demise in Alzheimer's dementia were more severe than those seen in the senile dementia affecting older people. Neurologists claimed there were behavioral differences, too: more restlessness and wandering in Alzheimer's, for example (possibly, it has turned out, because younger patients are generally healthier and can survive longer with their disease, giving it more time to wreak havoc).

Thus, in the opinion of most experts, Alzheimer's disease was a rare condition of the relatively young. In 1941, W. H. McMenemey, a British neuropathologist, wrote that "it would seem best to regard Alzheimer's disease as a psychosis of middle age which has a histological picture similar to but usually more extensive and severe than that of senile dementia." He added, "We are, as yet, entirely in the dark as to the nature of [the causative factors]; we conjecture that they are toxic or degenerative in origin, producing results in the [brain tissue] similar to those which we associate with a type of dementia found in the elderly." However, he wrote, "the last word remains to be said on the relationship of these diseases to one another."

Meanwhile, in America, people were living longer, and dementia rates were soaring. By the middle of the twentieth century, tens of thousands of elderly patients with dementia were living in mental asylums in the United States. In 1946, Congress created the National Institute of Mental Health to conduct research into dementia and other psychiatric disorders. Over the next two decades, thousands of demented patients were transferred out of decaying mental institutions and into nursing homes. Yet medicine still did not have a clear idea of what afflicted them.

Nevertheless, in the early 1970s, a consensus began to emerge that Alzheimer's disease (still believed to affect only middle-aged patients) and senile dementia (affecting the elderly) were, in fact, the same disease. In 1976, Robert Katzman, a decorated professor of neurology at the Albert Einstein College of Medicine in the Bronx, published a highly influential editorial in the *Archives of Neurology* arguing that distinctions between the two diseases were arbitrary. "Although further studies are indicated," he wrote, "the fact remains that neither the clinician, the neuropathologists, nor the electron microscopist can distinguish between the two disorders, except by the age of the patient."

Reviewing data from Europe, Katzman contended that potentially 1 million or more Americans were living with Alzheimer's disease. He calculated that between sixty thousand and ninety thousand Americans died of the disease every year—as loss of brain function leads to pneumonia, other infections from becoming bedridden, or loss of the ability to swallow, for example—making it the fourth or fifth most common cause of death in the United States, a fact ignored in standard tables of vital statistics. Katzman wrote, "The death certificates of patients with senile dementia bear witness to the bronchopneumonia, myocardial infarct, pulmonary embolus, cerebrovascular accident, or other acute event occurring at death. Such events may also mercifully end the life of patients with [cancer]. Yet, the latter diagnosis enters the death certificate as the first cause of death while we officially ignore the existence of senile dementia." He concluded: "We believe it is time to drop the arbitrary age distinction and adopt the single designation, Alzheimer disease."

If Katzman wanted to convince people that Alzheimer's disease was a widespread and deadly public health problem, he succeeded. In the span of just a few years, Alzheimer's went from being considered a relatively rare condition to being recognized as the fourth leading cause of death among the elderly in America.* In 1979 a group of families met in Chicago to start the Alzheimer's Association, a national advocacy group. In due course, Congress was spurred to establish a National Institute on Aging, which in 1984 created six national Alzheimer's Disease Research Centers to investigate basic mechanisms of the disease. In the 1980s and 1990s, public awareness only deepened as celebrities such as Rita Hayworth and Ronald Reagan were noted to be suffering from the disease. (Reagan's cognitive problems were already obvious in his second term.) Since then, federal funding for dementia research has increased to more than $3 billion, an almost eightfold rise since 2011. However, this outlay is still less than 50 percent of the research dollars we spend on cancer.

---

* According to Medline, only forty-two papers published in 1975 included "Alzheimer" as a keyword.

Today we recognize that there are several different types of dementia, of which Alzheimer's is the most common. Alzheimer's cases usually appear in old age, though 1 to 2 percent of cases occur in younger patients (like Auguste Deter) and are primarily hereditary in origin. Alzheimer's has a long gestation; the plaques and tangles that are a hallmark of the disease are believed to form more than a decade before cognitive impairment takes hold. So, in November 2014, when my father first visited Dr. Gordon, significant, probably irreversible, cellular and synaptic damage had already occurred in his brain.

Alzheimer's can affect many different brain regions. It often begins in the hippocampus, where long-term memory is processed, but the disease may also start in the temporoparietal lobes, causing language deficits, or in the frontal lobes, resulting in poor judgment or disinhibited behavior. Whatever the initial insult, the pathology spreads like wildfire. In the latter stages of the disease, patients' deficits are often very similar.

Drugs approved to treat the condition, such as Aricept, mostly treat symptoms, like memory loss (and even then with only minimal effectiveness). They do nothing to slow or reverse the progression of the disease. In 2021, the U.S. Food and Drug Administration approved the anti-amyloid drug aducanumab, though a panel of experts it had assembled objected.* Aducanumab and drugs like it target and

---

* In 2019, Biogen, the company that makes aducanumab, terminated a pair of late-stage studies of the drug after concluding that it produced no more benefit than a placebo. However, a few months later, the company unexpectedly resurrected the drug after analyzing a larger dataset that purportedly showed that aducanumab did indeed reduce cognitive decline in patients with early Alzheimer's who received higher doses.

The panel advising the FDA emphatically rejected this interpretation of the data, quashing not only the hopes of patients but also in some ways the very rationale of the prevailing research program. The rationale that removing clumps of beta-amyloid from patients' brains will result in better clinical outcomes had been the

eliminate amyloid plaques, which might be expected to slow Alzheimer's if amyloid is the principal cause of brain damage in the disease. However, anti-amyloid drugs have produced no reliably confirmed clinical benefit to date (and in some cases have worsened cognitive performance). If a drug can clear amyloid without producing significant clinical benefit, it is reasonable to assume that pathology other than amyloid must be a major cause of brain damage in dementia. Drugs targeting tau tangles are just now being studied.

As we move forward in dementia research, it is becoming clear that the dogma that Alzheimer's is just plaques and tangles must give way to a broader conceptualization of the disease. It could be that neither plaques nor tangles cause Alzheimer's; rather, they may simply be the by-products of another pathological process, such as inflammation. Recent evidence suggests that overactivity of brain immune cells called *microglia*, which devour unfamiliar pathogens and dead brain tissue, may accelerate brain degeneration. "The microglia become killers, not just janitors," Rudolph Tanzi, a prominent dementia researcher, has said. Several research groups and companies are trying to figure out how to influence genes that control inflammatory microglial activity. Indeed, small studies of anti-inflammatory drugs have shown some benefit in reducing the risk of developing Alzheimer's. Other research suggests that infectious agents, such as herpes viruses or the bacteria causing gum disease, may play a role in initiating amyloid buildup. These hypotheses may open new avenues of inquiry and treatment, including the use of antibiotics.

However, by the time most patients are diagnosed, so much cell death has already occurred that treating plaques or tangles will not

---

basis of Alzheimer's drug research for several decades. But accumulating evidence from aducanumab and other drug trials has called this hypothesis into question and argues for a reappraisal of the approach medical science has taken in dealing with the dementia epidemic.

result in any significant benefit. Thus, new research programs are focusing on growing neurons and restoring the synaptic connections between them.

Whatever happens in the future, it remains a fact that over the past four decades, hundreds of dementia drugs have fallen into the waste heap of failed Alzheimer's therapies. Dementia remains the only chronic and widespread medical scourge for which there are no effective treatments. What we can offer patients today has changed little from what Alzheimer was able to offer Auguste Deter in 1901. Faced with such a barren therapeutic landscape, patients and their families must summon extraordinary resilience.

7

THESE DAYS HAVE FINALLY COME

As my father's memory declined, so did my mother's movement and balance. Her disease progressed side by side with his, just as her life had for fifty years. She broke her foot in a fall and spent half a day in the emergency room. She suffered staring spells when she would become unresponsive, causing a new round of panic. More than once we took her to the ER to rule out stroke. She started having delusions, too, accusing my father of having paramours on Facebook. He laughed at first, but as the allegations persisted, he became despondent. "If after all these years you think I am going with girls, then I should drown myself," he said. Eventually, she required a live-in aide to help her with the basic activities of daily living: bathing, feeding, walking, dressing. She said to me, "Son, do the things you want when you are young. The decline will happen faster than you realize."

To manage her symptoms, we added more and different medications—fludrocortisone for low blood pressure, Seroquel for hallucinations, drugs to treat the side effects of other drugs—with little benefit, never knowing whether our mother would have been better off if we hadn't adjusted the medications in the first place. Even as Parkinson's robbed her of the life she'd enjoyed, a full life raising three successful children and managing a household that was always running on overdrive, my mother never asked, "Why me?" But we always said, "Why her?"

After each stepwise decline, she would insist, "If I can stay like this, it will be okay." She was able to recalibrate her expectations as her condition deteriorated, leaving her spirit mostly intact. But it was painful to watch. One day in early spring 2016 my brother, ever the pragmatist, said he wished our mother would die quickly. That was how our maternal grandfather had died, of a myocardial infarction just after his eighty-third birthday, and I remembered my mother had been grateful for the quick and painless demise. But I tore into my brother. I wasn't ready to lose my mother. I wanted her to remain alive for as long as possible.

At dinner at her home two weeks later, she told Rajiv's wife, Vandana, that the end was near. She spoke matter-of-factly, with the unvarnished bluntness of someone who has no more energy to waste on being diplomatic. There was an outpouring of tears, of course, but no real surprise. By then my mother could hardly get out of her recliner. I've learned over the years that patients often have a sixth sense about their deaths. They may have a feeling of impending doom before a heart attack or a fatal infection, for example, and though doctors don't know how to explain it, most of us take it seriously. That night, however, I ignored my mother's premonition. I told her not to worry. But she wasn't worried. She'd often said she didn't want to outlive my father. She was going to get her wish.

The morning she died about three weeks later, Rajiv called me from his car just before eight o'clock. It was an odd hour for him to be calling—I was getting ready to go to work—so I knew something was wrong. "Mom isn't doing well," he said calmly. "I think you should go over there."

I told him I would go after dropping my kids off at school.

"Go now," he said. "I think Mom just died."

It was a sunny April day. A mild breeze was blowing under a light blue, nearly cloudless sky. Speeding down the road, I called my father. He answered the phone coolly, but when he heard my voice, he started sobbing. He couldn't tell me anything—other than to drive carefully—so I told him to hand the phone to Harwinder, my mother's new aide. Harwinder told me that she had been awakened at five o'clock in the morning by groans. She called to my mother from her cot across the room, but my mother did not respond. She was about to get up to check on her when my mother took three deep breaths and went silent. She assumed my mother had gone back to sleep, but later in the morning when she tried to wake her, my mother did not react. She was not breathing; her skin was pale and cold. "She has completed, sir," Harwinder said before I heard my father shout that an ambulance had pulled up outside.

I had visited my mother only the night before. She was having a harder time walking than usual, slowly making her way back from the treadmill, where my father was still making her walk under supervision twice a day. When I asked how she was feeling, she admitted to some mild pressure on the left side of her chest, which I attributed to a recent fall. Now, maddeningly stuck on the road behind a school bus, I realized that the chest pain had probably been coronary angina, and that my mother had probably died of a heart attack in her sleep. Her heart, it appeared, had shown her a kind of mercy that her brain would not.

When I pulled up to my parents' house, there were no cars in the driveway. I ran up to the front door, but found it locked. I frantically rang the doorbell to no avail. When I called my brother, he told me the medics had taken my mother to the Plainview Hospital emergency room a couple of miles away. Rajiv had arrived just in time to prevent them from intubating her in the back of the ambulance. They had insisted on it—my mother's do-not-resuscitate form was in my brother's safe at home—but my brother was adamant, even pulling rank with his hospital ID. He was not going to let them assault our mother. It was plain to see, my brother told them, that she was gone.

In the ER I was led to a curtained-off space where Rajiv, Harwinder, and my father were sitting with my mother. She lay on a gurney, a purple throw draped over her. She had on red nail polish; a bright red bindi, signifying that she was married, still adorned her forehead. My father, his face swollen, sat on a stool beside the stretcher, his arms thrown over her body, his head resting on her arm. He touched her hands, massaged her feet. He asked Rajiv to take one last picture of them together, "for a memory," but my brother, broken up himself, would not. So I took the photograph. My parents' hands are clasped together, my mother's bone white, a red box of tissues in the space between them. Her mouth is open. My father asked me if they would close her mouth for the funeral. "She was so pretty," he said, and then he broke down.

In the wet, flat days that followed, there was so much to do—informing friends and relatives, receiving guests, arranging for the funeral and the cremation—that there was almost no time to grieve. But once the logistics were handled, I was pelted by grief. It would recede periodically only to hit me once again. At the funeral of a friend's mother two years before, a colleague had said to me, "You never really grow up until your parents die." Now, finally, I understood what he meant. What he meant was, while your parents are alive, there is always someone who thinks of you as a child. When I was a boy, my mother used to tell me a Hindu myth about a man who had been promised the world—unlimited riches—if he would just drown his mother. At the river, as he starts to submerge her in the frigid water, she implores, "Stay out of the water, Son! You will catch a cold."

It was raining on the day of the funeral. The mortuary, one of only two on Long Island with a crematorium, was about twenty miles east of Hicksville in the town of Ronkonkoma, on a small plot of land across the street from a strip mall. When my father and I arrived that morning, a light rain was drizzling my windshield. The treetops were shrouded in a cottony fog. "These days have finally come," he said before we left the car.

In the parlor, my mother's coffin lay among white flower bouquets shimmering in a milky light. Her body was dressed in her favorite silk salwar kameez. Inside the casket was one of the blankets I had found in the guest room the night she had been crying. "This will all be left behind," my father had said that day just three months earlier. And now, here we were.

The tragic absurdity of having two parents with brain diseases living and enduring with one another had finally come to a conclusion. Their diseases—his of the mind, hers of the flesh—were complementary, opposites, but like their owners made from the same stuff in the end.

The ceremony took about forty minutes. The pandit instructed my brother and me—and, at our insistence, our sister, though it did not conform with tradition—to repeat Sanskrit prayers and throw rice, water, and other provisions into a fire to sustain my mother in her journey into the afterlife. There was standing room only: scores of friends had come from across the country, especially from Fargo, to pay their respects. My father greeted them flatly, passively, but at times almost cheerfully. In those moments I found myself wondering if his damaged brain had taken away his capacity to properly grieve. The most painful thing I remember from that day is taking him aside to tell him to be sad, scolding him to give proper respect to this greatest of all losses.

After the service was over, Rajiv and I, our brother-in-law, Vini, and Rajiv's wife's brother, Gautam, serving as pallbearers, carried the lacquered wooden coffin out back, behind the white-shingled main building, to the crematorium. We put the box down on a gantry. The steel door of the incinerator was opened as the priest loudly chanted.

Inside the burner, I could see the blue flames licking at the metal grate. Men from the funeral home hoisted the casket off the platform. My father, now weeping, looked on as they stepped over to the burner and, without further ceremony, slid the casket into the blaze.

But then, as they started to close the door, he suddenly rushed grief-stricken toward the furnace and had to be held back by the shocked crowd from crawling into the fire with my mother.

PART II

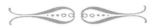

SCARS

8

YOU WANT TO PUT HIM IN A LOCKED UNIT
LIKE HIS MOTHER?

My mother's ashes remained in my parents' closet for almost two months. We couldn't decide whether to scatter them in the holy water at Haridwar, on the bank of the Ganges River in India; or in the Atlantic Ocean off the shore of Long Island. In the end, we elected not to make the long journey. So Rajiv booked a motorboat in Freeport, about ten miles southwest of Hicksville, and we set off on a bright morning just after Memorial Day to submerge my mother's remains. On the boat, the priest opened a suitcase and arranged the items we would need: incense, cotton balls, the urn, a few edibles. My father, dressed in brown slacks and a yellow shirt, watched impassively. He had never been particularly religious, and I hoped that for him the brunt of my mother's passing, after two difficult months and notwithstanding this last ritual, was finally over.

His response to her death had changed over the prior two months, becoming more automatic—"She was a good woman," "It is a big loss"—as if the memory of the trauma had been replaced by memories of that memory, which were themselves fading. For more than a year his memories of his life had been becoming generic, disconnected from time and place. He still remembered certain facts—that my mother was afraid of dogs, for example—but he had forgotten the specific events that led him to know these things. This shift from specific to general memories is typical as people age, owing to normal changes in the hippocampus, the part of the brain that—as the case of Henry Molaison showed—is required for both the laying down and the upkeep of specific memories. Elderly people may remember that they used to go camping when they were children, for instance, even if they do not remember specific experiences that occurred at a particular date and place. With Alzheimer's disease, in which the hippocampus is commonly damaged first, this process is often exaggerated. Eventually, as the disease spreads to the cortex, general memories also fade.

The pandit started off by draping long pieces of red thread over my brother's head and mine. He smeared tikkas of red paste on our brows. Next, he lit incense sticks and cotton balls soaked in oil. Rajiv and I made sixteen balls of dough about the size of a donut hole from flour, water, and milk and placed them on a metal plate, along with acorns, rice, and an assortment of seeds and other provisions—including holy water from Haridwar—that were supposed to sustain my mother in her final journey. As the boat sped hard over the waves, my belly churned. I had to keep my waist in contact with the priest's table to keep from falling over. The priest unscrewed the top of the urn, and we sprinkled holy water on the plastic bag containing my mother's remains. We then opened the bag and poured in more water and some milk, along with the items on the plate. Next, we emptied the contents of the bag into a white wicker basket. The ashes were charcoal gray; it was hard to believe that this was all that was left of her body. We placed the empty plastic bag in the basket, too. Then we waited for the dust to settle.

The boat slowed to a stop. As the eldest son, Rajiv was given the honor of scattering the ashes, but I would not have been able to do so anyway; by then I was feeling horribly seasick. While the priest chanted, his bald pate glistening in the summer heat, Rajiv placed the wicker basket with my mother's remains on a metal hook at the end of a long pole. Then, without ceremony or words—apart from the Sanskrit syllables spitting out from the priest's lips—he leaned over the side of the boat and lowered the basket into the water. It had a metal weight to help it sink. My father, sitting on a bench along the railing, squinted in the sunlight watching the basket submerge, its contents exploding into a murky cloud in the greenish water. The priest told us to clasp our hands together in prayer. No one said anything as he violently chanted. Then, when he was done, a crew member retrieved the basket with some rope and lifted it back on board. The boat turned around to head back to shore.

My father rode with me on the way home. We were both tired, and my stomach was just beginning to settle. I put on Beethoven's Piano Sonata no. 8, the *Pathétique*, and looked over at my father. He was staring ahead quietly, listening to the music. I rolled down the window, and a hot wind passed over us. He said nothing for a while; there were only the shrieks and wails of passing cars. Then he said, "We spent our whole life together. I miss her all the time."

I took my father to a bereavement group organized through my hospital, but he stopped going after two sessions. He had little in common with the other participants, he told me. But the real reason, I believe, was that he was uninterested in taking even the smallest steps to get on with his life. To him, it was a distinctly American concept: "moving on," starting over, remaking yourself, even after your faithful partner of almost fifty-one years has passed away. The woman he'd criticized and browbeaten into compliance for the past year and a half was now elevated to mythic status. His memories—such as they were—omitted the last few years of her decline and retained only earlier, happier remembrances of the patient and modest woman who had stuck by his side—not so different, it turned out, from my own memories of my mother. Her pictures adorned every table and wall in the house. They were right there in front of him, no matter where he turned, so he could stare at her smiling face as he watched TV or picked disinterestedly at the meals my mother's aide, Harwinder, who had agreed to stay on temporarily, prepared but could not get him to eat.

That spring was a lonely time. Friends and relatives who had reached out in the wake of my mother's death largely disappeared. Part of the reason for this was that my father had never been especially social. As a beneficiary of his spouse's amiability, he had done little to develop friendships or rectify his faults. When my mother died, so too did he, it seemed, at least in people's minds. It didn't help that he lacked social graces. He had always done things the wrong way: mowing the lawn at night, waking the neighbors; bringing up controversial subjects like Kashmiri separatism at low-key social gatherings. When we were kids, he used to trim our nails with a Gillette razor blade, twisting our fingers painfully so they wouldn't get lacerated. As long as the nails got cut, it didn't matter to my father how much we protested. That sort of encapsulated his personality: disciplined, unsentimental, focused solely on the task at hand.

My mother used to affectionately call him *poottha*, awkward. But after she was gone, the rest of the world was not so forgiving. As a widower, my father found himself alone much of the time. He would watch Indian television, go on short walks, and take frequent naps. Once a week I would take him out to lunch or dinner, and every month or so to my kids' school functions. But with my mother no longer his companion, these outings did not hold much appeal anymore. Sometimes they hardly seemed to register in his brain. I remember an evening that May, about six weeks after my mother's funeral, when

I took my father to Pia's spring concert. After the concert, we were heading up to his bedroom when he stopped me. He asked me when Pia's concert was. He was looking forward to it.

Unfortunately, my father became cognitively impaired in what the bioethicist Stephen Post and others have called a hypercognitive world. In this world swirling with information, we prioritize intellect and reason as the predominant virtues. If you do not possess these virtues, you are marginalized. If you cannot follow or add to the endless conversation, you are rendered invisible. "We live in a culture that is the child of rationalism and capitalism," Post wrote in *The Moral Challenge of Alzheimer Disease*, "so clarity of mind and economic productivity determine the value of human life." The writer Kent Russell wrote of the way "the world spins faster and faster until those who used to be a part of it [get] separated, like sediment in a centrifuge." This is what happened to my father as his brain degenerated. Unable to maintain friendships, respect social cues, or bond over shared history, he became largely invisible to the outside world.

As we've noted, Tom Kitwood, the British social psychologist, wrote about "malignant" social environments that, through either implicit messaging or explicit neglect, diminish an impaired person's personhood. Such environments are common in Western cultures, in which independence and individualism are generally celebrated, but they are present, too, in other cultures in which the elderly are seemingly more venerated. In some African countries, for example, dementia is blamed on witchcraft, and those living with it may be shunned or persecuted. In Colombia, the condition is called La Bobera, or "the foolishness," and is often attributed to omens or other superstitious causes. In China, the name for Alzheimer's roughly translates as "elderly retardation" or "brain regression" disease. To exist with dementia in such a world means to live condemned.

Sadly, the social isolation that often results for patients is associated with accelerated cognitive decline. A few months after my mother died I read a 2007 paper, "Loneliness and Risk of Alzheimer Disease," published in the *Archives of General Psychiatry*, that studied 823 people initially free of dementia who were recruited from churches, social services agencies, and senior citizen facilities in and around Chicago. To assess their degree of loneliness, the researchers asked the participants to fill out a five-item questionnaire, agreeing or disagreeing with statements such as "I miss having people around," "I often feel abandoned," and "I miss having a really good friend."

Participants were assessed in other ways, too: how often they interacted with their social network; how often they exercised or participated in cognitively stimulating activities, such as reading; and how often they said they felt sad or depressed. Their cognitive function was evaluated regularly by trained psychiatrists. Those who died underwent autopsy to evaluate the degree of brain damage, including strokes, amyloid plaques, and tau tangles.

The researchers found that in the seventy-six subjects who developed Alzheimer's disease, the risk of the condition was twice as high in the loneliest persons as compared with those who had the most social support, even after controlling for cognitive and physical activity. This association did not depend on race, income, level of disability, or the presence of vascular risk factors. Neuropathology, the researchers concluded, is not the sole driver of clinical Alzheimer's.

This study had limitations, of course—the participants were predominantly white and were observed for an average of only three years. Yet the conclusion was inescapable: more frequent social activity is associated with lower dementia risk.

Consistent with these findings, I learned that autopsy studies have shown that brain damage (i.e., plaque or tangle volume) and degree of clinical dementia are not as strongly correlated as one might expect. Patients with only a small amount of brain damage often have "excess disability" out of proportion to their neurological impairment. The converse is also true: patients with a large amount of plaques and tangles may be surprisingly cognitively intact. The usual explanation for this discrepancy is "cognitive reserve"—higher educational levels, prior intelligence, and so on—but what is rarely acknowledged is the vital role of "psychosocial reserve"—relationships, environment, and family support—which studies have shown may be just as important as neuropathology.

The kind of loneliness my father experienced after my mother's death is considered especially detrimental. In a paper published in 2020 in the *Journal of the American Medical Association*, researchers for the Harvard Aging Brain Study studied 257 cognitively unimpaired men and women whose brains had a high density of beta-amyloid plaques as measured by PET scans. After adjusting for factors such as age, sex, socioeconomic status, and amyloid levels, they found that over a span of three years, participants who were widowed experienced mental decline that was three times faster than that of similar people who had not lost a spouse. Furthermore, widowed participants who had the highest baseline amyloid plaque levels exhibited the steepest decline, suggesting that widowhood and beta-amyloid combined may compound the risk of cognitive impairment.

Indeed, we know that the chronic stress that occurs in a state of widowhood and social isolation strongly impairs brain function. The hippocampus, for example, is especially sensitive to cortisol, a stress hormone: high levels of cortisol can interfere with both short-term memory and its transfer into long-term storage. Repeated exposure to stress hormones has also been shown to cause atrophy and scarring in the hippocampus and the prefrontal cortex (which controls working memory) in both rats and humans. Such stress may also induce neuroinflammation, along with plaques and tangles.

All of this is to say that my father's social isolation may have been not just a consequence of his dementia but also a cause. Pathways linking biology with social psychology run both ways. Psychology may reflect brain damage but can cause it as well.

Sadly, the malignant social psychology that caused my father to become isolated emanated from his family, too. I wish I could say that we were more patient than the world outside, but we weren't. The Etch A Sketch that was his mind trapped him in a perpetual present—and his children in perpetual frustration. I wish I could forget how we would scold him when he'd ask questions, telling him that it was pointless when he could not remember the answers. Sometimes my siblings and I would talk about him as if he weren't there. "He is helpless." "He won't remember." "He is like a child now." We would say those things in front of him, sometimes even *to* him. There was little to deter us, even as we regretted it, again and again, after the fact. We knew that our father was more than just his damaged brain. We knew it, but we struggled to believe it.

One morning that July, about three months after my mother died, the family was together at the house. Suneeta had flown in from Minneapolis the previous week to look at assisted-living facilities. She wanted a plan, she said, for my father's long-term care. Harwinder, my mother's aide, was staying on for the time being, but how long was she going to stick around? Her husband, sick with diabetes and kidney disease, and her extended family were in India.

A rotund and mostly jovial woman, Harwinder had come to the United States to work so she could send money back home. Like many working-class women from South Asia, she had chosen caregiving for the elderly, a reflection of the great demand for workers in this area but also of her culture, which demanded care and respect for elders. But my sister was worried about what was going to happen when Harwinder eventually went back to India. Where was my father going to live if we could not find proper help? These were some of the questions she had come to address.

That morning, Harwinder was in the kitchen making breakfast, while I was at the dining table, sorting through piles of my father's old papers. For weeks I had been wanting to throw out the countless documents and mementos he had amassed that he had no use for anymore—a burden, I often thought bitterly, my mother had had to endure her entire married life. The clutter for me had come to embody his scarred brain. We needed to get rid of it, I felt, to give him (and us) a new beginning.

"Rajiv is paying your bills now," I said, holding up an old phone receipt. "You can throw this out."

"Leave it," my father barked, trying to slap the paper out of my hand.

"Let him do it, Dad," Suneeta pleaded, realizing I was not going to back down this time. If Harwinder hadn't hurried in from the kitchen to usher my father upstairs for his late-morning nap, there would have been a full-blown row.

When my father was gone, I quickly began to fill up garbage bags, counting on the fact that he would forget the piles had been there when he woke up. Among the papers I threw out were old bank statements, old credit-card bills, printed copies of newspaper articles, and scientific reprints going back to the 1950s that could all be found online. In a way it was sad to see it go, this avalanche of cuttings and Xeroxes that had once been the measure of his life. Files on Mandela, Gandhi, and Martin Luther King; Einstein, Crick, and Barbara McClintock; Frederick Douglass and Rabindranath Tagore—my father's political, intellectual, and cultural heroes—soon poked out of white plastic bags. I'd once planned to clean up his papers after he died. But it was beginning to feel like he was already gone.

When I was done with a portion of the table, I went up to my father's study, the one room in the house he rarely entered anymore. I could still see him crouching over his desk, reeking of rubber cement, painstakingly preparing a figure for one of his monographs while my mother implored him to come for dinner. (She always said that nothing good or substantial would come from writing books.) On the Formica table were assorted reprints and micrographs. In a filing cabinet I found more decades-old Coldwell Banker statements, eviction notices on a small property he once owned, and more old papers and old bills. There were copies of an article he had published in the 1969 *Hindustan Times* on the future of biology. In a folder marked "Memories" I found notes dating back to about 2014, the year he retired, that he had written to himself about people he knew— "Retired long time ago"; "Still lives in the same house in Michigan"; "Theft in November"—inscribed in increasingly shaky handwriting. Contact information had proliferated, too, with copy after copy in folder after folder, as if he had been desperately trying to hold on to the information but had forgotten what he had already kept. All redundant copies went into the trash.

It was amazing to see the meticulous records he had kept. Nearly every conversation he'd ever had, it seemed, even the most insignificant, was recorded in handwritten notes. There was correspondence related to the issuance of his first driver's license in 1972. There were receipts for donations he had made to Indian orphanages over the years. There were copies of his favorite sayings (and copies of those copies). There were enough newspaper printouts to fill a library. He seemed to have had a special fascination with the pregnant Britney Spears.

There were troves of letters, too. Much of his scientific correspondence had been social: arranging meetings with colleagues at conferences, for example, or congratulating them on their accomplishments (while reminding them of his own). But scores of more serious letters were collected in red-lined folders under headings like "Exploitation of Foreign Scientists," "Intellectual Slavery," and "NAACP/EEOC." One, from an Indian scientist in 1980, three years after we arrived in America, encouraged my father to fight the unfair system that was denying him tenure: "Prem, we have talked about it earlier, but I would like to repeat it again: We have to fight, and fight fearlessly, for our rights. They say, faint heart never wins a fair lady, and this is applicable in our situation, too—unless we fight tooth and nail, nothing will be achieved."

Another letter, this one addressed to my mother, was from a scientist, Kathy, whom my father had worked with when he was on a research sabbatical in Berkeley.

> The two of you deserve so much more than you've received since arriving in this country, eager to belong. America is my home and, of course, I love it. It's a large and diverse country, marvelous and magnificent in so many ways. We have an extraordinary Constitution, written by ordinary people of vision, wisdom and humanity. All too often, though, bias and bigotry, fear, poverty and ignorance, dull the luster and rob the country of its vigor and promise.
>
> I do hope that [Prem's new job] will be the beginning of a happy, productive future. Hopefully, Prem will get the support and recognition he deserves for his work. Prem's persistence and determination, his pride and honesty, are quite exceptional. I'm certain that these, along with the devotion and support of a loving family, have given him the courage to continue to prevail. Still, when I saw him today, he seemed low, sad. I don't know whether it's the sadness that always comes when we must bid farewell to the past (no matter how bright the future). Or the sadness of regret. Regret for the lost time, for having had to cope with people who exploited him and treated him shabbily. I don't think I've heard Prem

give that uninhibited, delighted laugh of his since he learned that [another] position we thought he'd secured would not materialize. Hopefully, by Monday he'll be his usual optimistic self.

The letters brought back memories of how much my father's professional struggles had determined the atmosphere in our home growing up. We left India to advance his academic career, but in America he never achieved the kind of success he felt he deserved—denied for years, he believed, by a racist university tenure system that forced him to take postdoctoral positions with no long-term stability and left him embittered and in a constant state of conflict with professional colleagues. He learned to approach life's conundrums as if they were Aesopian fables. He adopted the habit of distilling life's problems into simple aphorisms dealing with faith, persistence, the value of work—Booker T. Washington stuff.

He was always saying things like "The happiest of people don't necessarily have the best of everything; they just make the most of everything that comes their way." Or he would say, "Success is measured not so much by the position one has reached in life as by the obstacles one has had to overcome." Or "Work is worship." Or "It is not falling in water but staying there that drowns a man." Or "I'm a tremendous believer in luck. I find that the harder I work, the more I have of it." (Or sometimes he would mangle the adage, as when he would say, "Don't change horses in the middle of the ocean.") He believed strongly in focus, determination—he'd written his first textbook in the back bedroom, littered with scientific papers and light micrographs, while working full-time as a postdoc—and also that the mind is malleable, that satisfaction is a state of mind. "The Ladder of St. Augustine," Longfellow's inspiring poem, had always graced his bedroom wall, and I found it again—several copies, in fact—in the piles in his now-defunct study:

The heights by great men reached and kept
Were not attained by sudden flight,
But they, while their companions slept,
Were toiling upward in the night.

In a desk drawer I found some old photographs in Kodak envelopes. There was a black-and-white picture of my parents as a young couple, probably newlyweds, posing together in a field in what appears to be a hill station, most likely Kashmir in northern India, gently kissing. It is a strange sight: I saw them kiss on the mouth only once in my entire life. Because they are standing on an incline, my father, looking impossibly short in slacks and a sport jacket, is bending down to touch my mother's lips. She is wearing a salwar kameez and a light cardigan, and has the demure, modest look of brides in old Bollywood movies. The landscape is scarred and barren; apart from a small barn in the distance, there is no sign of life. I stare at the photograph, wondering, Who was there to take this picture?

Another picture, overexposed or perhaps lightened by the years, is of us children playing in the snow at the cottage in Kentucky we moved into when we arrived in America in January 1977. My brother, wearing a T-shirt, brown jacket, and sneakers, is standing, cool-cat style, at the edge of our icy driveway. I am coming up behind him, carrying a snowball. My four-year-old sister, wearing a red winter coat, is giggling at our antics. My mother is sitting in the car in the driveway, the front passenger door open, probably scolding us for our shenanigans. The picture fills me with nostalgia, but there is something odd about it. Then it hits me: it is reversed. Wasn't the driveway on the other side?

Most of my memories of that house are of us being snowed in; it was an especially brutal winter that year in Kentucky. My sister and I shared a bedroom, while Rajiv slept on a folding bed in the dining room next to a clanging radiator, dozing off most nights to

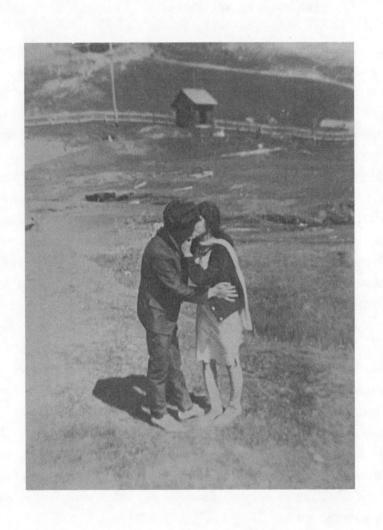

a University of Kentucky basketball game on his tiny transistor radio. We ate meals on a scuffed wooden table that doubled as a Ping-Pong table after Rajiv and I installed a makeshift net of twine secured by two pencils. When we received a rare phone call from India, my mother would automatically begin to wail, convinced she was going to receive the news that one of her parents had died. The house was always freezing, but I don't remember us ever complaining. We took my father at his word that President Carter had asked citizens to turn the thermostat down to fifty-five degrees Fahrenheit at night to ease the energy crisis.

In the following spring, my father tilled the half-acre plot in the back of the house by himself. He planted lettuce, red chilies, and tomatoes systematically marked with plastic labels jutting out of the fertile soil. Along the wooden fence separating us from our neighbor, he grew green beans and cucumbers, which spread wildly over the broken slats as if trying to find an escape. He planted beets and eggplant, too, till the garden was overrun and tendrils swallowed up any remaining patch of grass.

In the early evening we would stand side by side and water the plants. I took great pride in being there with him—being chosen to be there over my brother. When the watering was done, I would aim the hose skyward, waiting for the cold pellets to send a welcome shiver through my sweaty skin, while my father would yell at me to stop the foolishness.

Many of my memories of that year revolve around that backyard. There was a lawn mower whose engine imprinted a coin-sized burn on my thigh. There was a small woodshed that housed shovels, gardening tools, and various rusted hulks. And in the middle of the yard, there was a grand oak tree with a tire swing. I can still see my father sitting on a lawn chair under that tree—his fingers caked with soil, his cold beer trickling condensation—predicting how bounteous the harvest would be that fall.

He was right. My mother froze the vegetables, and we ate them through the autumn and winter. When school started my father would walk me to the bus stop every morning, just as he had in New Delhi. Then the snows came, and we had snowball fights on the lawn.

It is hard to believe that I still remember so many details from that time nearly five decades ago. Was the garden visible through the kitchen window? Was that window really framed by frilly white curtains? Memory construction, psychologists say, involves a tension between two opposing principles. *Correspondence* tries to force our memories to agree with the original event that we experienced. It is how most of us view memory: as a true reproduction of something that occurred in the past. The principle of *coherence*, on the other hand, transforms our memories to make them consistent with the way we see ourselves and the world in the present. Through coherence, our memories are reconstructed to support our current values or beliefs. These beliefs may not allow us to see things the way they really happened. Those kitchen curtains may now be white to reflect the nostalgia with which I reflect, forty-five years later, on my family's first year in America. Thus, autobiographical memories involve a balance of two conflicting forces, one aiming to represent the past the way it was, the other aiming to reconstruct the past in the way that we need to see it today.

"He put me through hell last week," my brother said. I looked up from where I was sitting at the table, sorting through our family's old photos. "First, he accused me of stealing Mom's jewelry. Then he went missing. Went out on his own to H&Y Marketplace and got lost. Harwinder freaked out. Then he locked the bathroom door from the outside, so I had to come over to open it. He couldn't use his computer twice, so I had to come over for that, too. Complete torture."

"I wonder if we should ask his neighbor to help with these issues and tell him that we would pay him for his time," I said.

"Sandeep, Dad doesn't even feel comfortable with you doing things for him, how will he with anyone else? He just calls me. And honestly, I am tired."

"So, don't make yourself so available," I said, feeling irritated by my brother's typically boastful self-pity.

"I've tried," Rajiv replied. "He calls me incessantly. I had to come here at nine p.m. because he couldn't check his emails, which I set up with a single click. He forgot the password: Raj. Then, instead of being grateful, he accused me of fucking up his email account."

"Well, don't take it so personally," I said, crumpling a piece of paper. "He has dementia."

"Just because he has dementia doesn't mean he can't act like a dick," my brother shot back.

Harwinder, carrying a basket of freshly laundered clothes, came up from the basement. She turned and went upstairs to fold the clothes.

"It breaks my heart, but he needs a different kind of care," my sister said. "Not some local women we find through ads in *India Abroad*."

Suneeta had been visiting assisted-living facilities over the previous week. One she liked called the Atria, in nearby Glen Cove, had an impressive array of amenities: one- and two-bedroom apartments, a movie theater, a game room, and an on-site salon. Nurses were on duty twenty-four hours a day. Housekeeping was provided, too, along with prepared meals. But it was expensive, about $9,000 a month for what my sister wanted, and since my father didn't have long-term care insurance, we would have to pay for it out of pocket. He had savings and a government pension, which would cover most of it. But the remainder, my sister informed us, would be split among the three of us.

"I think it's the best option," she said as I sifted through another pile of papers. "I realized when I did the math last week that I didn't add in the cost of someone staying with him at night, which we'll eventually need if Harwinder only wants to work during the day." She made some rough calculations. At $150 a night, the cost of night-time help would be about $4,500 a month. We were already paying Harwinder $130 per day, six days a week, so if we got her to agree to seven days, the total outlay for twenty-four-hour, privately hired care would be about $8,400 a month, plus food and tips. "So, in the end, it's about the same as assisted living," my sister concluded. "I mean, if I'm missing something, tell me."

"I don't think we should worry about the money part," Rajiv said. "Dad should be at ease in his final stages."

"And this is being at ease?" I said drily. "You want to put him in a locked unit like his mother?"

"Of course not," my sister cried, "but this"—she waved her arms—"is no solution. Once Harwinder leaves, we will have to find someone else. Then that person leaves, and again we're in the same boat."

"She's right," Rajiv said. "We've had four people stay less than a day."

"With assisted living we never have to worry about someone leaving," Suneeta went on. "Sure, it's a bit more money, but if we put our foot down, I'm sure we can convince Dad." Her eyes searched the room frantically.

"He needs Indian food," I blurted out.

"Fuck Indian food," my sister responded. "What's more important, Indian food or peace of mind? You guys can bring him Indian food twice a week."

I picked up the trash bags I'd filled and went to the front door.

"Look, I leave in a couple of days," Suneeta said, "so I want this resolved before I go. I don't see Harwinder leaving anytime soon, but we should decide: if she leaves, what do we do with Dad, and if his memory gets worse, what do we do? It doesn't hurt to have a plan."

I opened the front door. It was a scalding day. A few American flags were still flying for the Fourth of July, but nothing was stirring in the stale, still air. I hauled the garbage bags out to the curb and threw them into a pile on the grassy island at the edge of the sidewalk. Then I pulled the brochures for the Atria assisted-living facility and the director's business card from my shorts pocket and inserted them into one of the bags. I got into my car. It had been a long morning. I would do the rest of the cleaning another day.

9

SHE TOLD ME SHE WILL WORK FOR FREE

That autumn, on a trip to the Netherlands to give a book talk, I visited a nursing home about ten miles southeast of Amsterdam, in the small town of Weesp. The Hogeweyk, as it is called, pioneered a radically innovative model of dementia care when it opened in 2009. It was built as a "dementia village," in which its 150 or so residents, most with advanced disease requiring around-the-clock support, could wander freely through the facility's buildings and outdoor spaces, albeit under the watchful eye of cameras and caregivers. In the past decade, versions of the facility have sprung up in France, Canada, and the United States. Though I didn't expect that my father would be moving to an institutional setting anytime soon, I was hoping to learn more about what novel assisted-living arrangements could offer.

From the train station in Weesp I walked about a mile through the sleepy town, past utilitarian apartment complexes and stately homes with docks along a canal. It was a chilly, desolate day. A man was quietly working in his garden, but the only human sounds I heard were children playing at a preschool.

At the entrance to the facility I was greeted by Leo, one of the founders of The Hogeweyk and now a senior consultant. A handsome, earnest man in his early fifties, dapperly dressed that day in a gray business suit, he took me on a quick walk through the village—down the main street, through a large courtyard (the "town square"), past the fountain, and into an indoor mall, where we sat down at the café for a chat. Soft jazz was playing on the stereo. Leo ordered sparkling water for himself and a Diet Coke for me. "Every day is different," he said as I peered out the window onto mostly empty walkways. "Yesterday, people were milling around. Today it is frigid, and people are staying indoors."

The residents of the village, he told me, live in twenty-three individual houses, in six- or seven-person "families," each with a trained caretaker. "We wanted a family structure because that is how humans want to live, with a few other people with similar interests and mindsets," he said. He and his cofounders asked themselves what they would want for their own parents if they developed dementia and needed long-term care. The answer they came up with was homes where their parents could develop friendships with like-minded companions. "The house is a recognizable system," he told me. "Not like a memory ward where people sit in the same chair for hours."

I couldn't help but remember the ward at the Elim Rehab and Care Center in Fargo, where my paternal grandmother, my Mataji, Maya, spent the last two years of her life before her death in 1994. Mataji, a widow by the age of forty-five, was a resolute woman who ruled the roost (and her daughter-in-law, my mother) until she lost her mind. We used to visit her at the first-floor memory unit that would become her final home. She'd be sitting, stooped, in a circle of wheelchairs, a thin white scarf over her head, semiconsciously passing beads through her spindly fingers while she muttered prayers. I hated the place: the ceramic floors, the nauseating smell of disinfectant, the cries of the residents being force-fed medicated pudding. It all reeked of shit and hopelessness. But my parents would visit every day, bringing fruits and a sort of patronizing cheer to Mataji and the other unfortunate tenants. Having been raised in a culture in which old people are held in high regard—or at least not locked in dementia wards—my parents enjoyed the company of elders, though the sad irony of Mataji spending her last years in a nursing home always seemed lost on my father.

Leo told me that he had been a facilities manager at the old nursing home around which The Hogeweyk was built, on essentially the same four-acre plot of land. (The nursing home was then demolished.) Despite the sophisticated amenities, the new facility operates on basically the same budget as any traditional nursing home in the Netherlands: about €6,000 a month per person, much of it subsidized by the Dutch government. "Six thousand per patient?" I asked. "Per *resident*," Leo corrected. But the outlay is spent differently, he emphasized. "Much more is possible for the same amount of money," he said.

Before residents are placed into a house, they and their families are interviewed about the kind of life they have led, their habits and values, and what they want from the life ahead. "We want to know your background, your preferred lifestyle," Leo said, gesturing up and down with his hands to convey balance. "Dutch food or international cuisine. Local news versus world news. We provide choices."

The village touts a model of dementia care called *reminiscence therapy*, which attempts to recreate the kind of daily life residents were familiar with before they started to lose their memories. The idea is to hone the spirit and architecture of the village's homes to reflect the lifestyle the residents were accustomed to in their younger days. One universal characteristic of autobiographical memory is the *reminiscence bump*, the retention of memories for events that occurred between the ages of ten and thirty, usually the most influential years in a person's life. Milestone events in these years—schooling, the gaining of independence, marriage—are often remembered, even by people living with dementia. These memories, and the environment in which they were made, can be used to sustain a sense of identity.

There used to be seven lifestyles represented among the village's houses, but now there are only four, all for the same price. In "haute bourgeois" houses, in which the residents are often upper class or well-to-do, manners are more proper, and residents tend to go to bed later and sleep into the morning. Classical music is often played, and the cuisine is more French than traditional Dutch. By contrast, in "urban" houses the music is more contemporary. Walls may be painted in kitschy pink, and the residents usually prefer beer to wine. The "craftsman" lifestyle accommodates residents who once might have been laborers or worked in small family businesses or on farms. They tend to wake up earlier in the morning as they might have done when they worked in the fields. The décor is plain, the residents tend to listen to folk music, and meals are traditional, involving lots of potatoes and nothing too exotic. The "cultural" lifestyle is designed for residents who once loved to travel and had—or perhaps still have—a deep interest in art and music.

During the day, residents can wander about as in any neighborhood, watched over by the 250 or so caregivers who staff the supermarket and the hair salon, take care of the gardens, and so on. They can go out to the pub and have a beer. They can sit on a bench by the pond and watch the ducks or passersby. If they get lost, there is always someone around who will help them get home. (There is only one door in and out of the facility.) The founders, Leo told me, believed people would want to exchange some safety for freedom, a fraught trade-off in eldercare. "People said, 'What if they climb over the railing and fall in the fountain?'" he said, scoffing. "Well, people with dementia are not stupid. They don't jump over a fence into a pond."

Though the residents sometimes go on special day trips to shopping malls or to nearby towns, much of a typical day revolves around preparing and consuming the evening meal. Residents can accompany the house caretaker to the supermarket to shop for ingredients. They can help prepare the meal, too—stirring sauces, chopping vegetables, etc.—as much as they want and are able to. Or they can sit back and enjoy the smells of the meal being prepared, as in any normal home. The caretakers, all with at least three years of specialized dementia and geriatric training, endeavor to keep the residents engaged while still doing the work of a regular house.

As we talked, I noticed an elderly woman dressed in gray slacks and a dark gray coat, sitting by herself at a nearby table. She was originally from Senegal, Leo told me, and had been coming by herself to the café since her husband, who'd also lived at The Hogeweyk, had passed away recently. On our way out, we stopped by her table to say hello. "Go ahead and ask her a few questions," Leo said encouragingly. The woman had a shock of gray hair, like a dandelion. I asked her how long she had lived at The Hogeweyk, but Leo immediately interrupted me. "That could be a difficult question," he said with a touch of rebuke. "Time is a difficult thing." Instead, he asked her in an open-ended way about how she was doing. She answered meanderingly, telling a story (I think) about chickens, perhaps ones she had lived with when she was a girl in West Africa. Leo listened patiently, nodding frequently. After we left, I asked him what the woman had meant. "I don't know," he replied.

We went for another walk. It was early evening by then, and the air was freezing. We passed by the reading club and ducked briefly into the Mozart room, with its gilt mirrors and period furniture and instruments. The amenities in the village were extraordinary, but I wondered whether the residents could appreciate the life that the facility was endeavoring to create—or rather recreate. Wasn't the model of care that Leo and others espoused undermined by the disease they were trying to manage? Before coming that day, I'd read complaints online that The Hogeweyk's amenities, often located at a substantial distance from the residential houses—as one would expect in a normal village—were largely inaccessible to residents unable to walk. If that were true, then wasn't the facility a sort of Potemkin village, intended mostly for the benefit of caregivers or visiting relatives and not, primarily, for the residents it was entrusted to care for?

Not surprisingly, Leo took exception to my question. "It is not fake," he said as he walked me to the exit. Residents did participate in the village's activities, he insisted, to the extent that they were able. Of course, some couldn't leave their homes, but they were likely to die soon anyway.

But, I persisted, what about the carefully curated homes, the caretakers posing as gardeners? Wasn't it all a stage set like in the movie *The Truman Show*, designed to convince residents of something that wasn't true—that they were at home, when actually they were far from their homes and would never be able to go back?

"That is not lying," Leo replied. "It is called therapeutic deception. It is dealing with dementia the way it is."

He went on: "If a patient is asking for her daughter, and you know the daughter isn't coming, you say, 'She will come in a couple of hours.'" It was better to validate a resident's perspective than to try again and again to reorient it, he explained. If a resident wanted to go home and you knew it wasn't possible, it was better to distract the person, even if it meant letting him wait at a "bus stop" till he got tired and forgot what he was waiting for.

"It is done for humanitarian reasons," Leo said, like telling children there is a Santa Claus. "Is that lying?" he asked rhetorically. "Of course not." He mentioned the U.S. president at the time. "Trump lives in his own reality, and we have come to accept it. Why can't we be as patient and accommodating with demented patients?"

By the time I got back to Central Station in Amsterdam, it was late, and I was tired. I stopped by a coffee shop and smoked a joint, then walked back to my hotel. The waterways were shimmering that evening. The annual winter light festival was going on, and elaborate displays illuminated the canals. As I wandered through the maze of cobblestone streets, I got lost. The streets were curved and met at funny angles. Try as I might, I still couldn't keep track of how they connected or where I had just been. One turn, and I would find myself at a place on the map that I couldn't imagine having gotten to, and I couldn't figure out where the lapse in reasoning had been. So—and the irony was not lost on me, even in my disoriented state—I stopped random people on the street to ask for help. I asked them to repeat themselves. I forgot what they told me and stopped someone else. After almost an hour, I finally made it back to my hotel. But the lights, the paintings, the glass sculptures along the way: they were spectacular.

Some years ago, the British Alzheimer's Society issued the following statement on therapeutic deception (or what some call "validation therapy"): "We struggle to see how systematically deceiving someone with dementia can be part of an authentic trusting relationship in which the person's voice is heard and their rights promoted." It was a subject over which my siblings and I often clashed. More pragmatic than I, they had no reservations about employing deception to help our father (and themselves) get through one of his rancorous moods. They would tell him what he wanted to hear. To them, telling the truth wasn't worth the trouble if it upset him.

But I fought against this practice. To me, a healthy relationship with our father, even in his debilitated state, could only be based on truth and trust. Little lies, even if told with the best of intentions, would erode what little connection we had left with him. I understood my siblings' motivation, of course. The biggest problem in caring for my father after my mother died wasn't his memory loss or repetitive questions as much as his behavior: the tantrums, verbal abuse, and sometimes violence. As we've noted, the human amygdala, responsible for the processing of emotions, is only a few millimeters from the hippocampus. Disease in one area travels quickly to the other, so amnesia often coexists with emotional outbursts out of proportion to the events that triggered them. Lies and deception were a shortcut to navigating such fraught moments. And what did a lie even mean when my father could hardly tell the difference between truth and falsehood or remember what had been said?

Yet lying, I still believed, was a poor strategy for dealing with my father, both on a moral and a practical level. He was already paranoid. He would accuse us of not being straight with him. He believed Rajiv was stealing his money. Our lies, if they were discovered, would only deepen his distrust. But more importantly, they eroded his dignity (and ours). They rendered him a person who was no longer worth reckoning with. To me, telling my father the truth, even if it was painful or provocative, was a gesture of respect. It was saying that we still thought of him as being a part of our world.

I came to this view from the perspective of a doctor as much as from that of a son. In medicine, historically, physicians have often deceived their patients. We used to withhold bad news, such as the diagnosis of a terminal illness. Such paternalism was once widely accepted in medicine. In the mid-nineteenth century, the American Medical Association's code of ethics stated that physicians have a "sacred duty" to "avoid all things which have a tendency to discourage the patient and depress his spirits." But times have changed. The prevailing ethical mantra in medicine is now patient autonomy. Today, patients have the right to direct their own care, and to do so they must be fully informed. As doctors, we no longer "care for" our patients through their illnesses as much as "care with" them.

Lying in dementia care, ironically, was frowned upon till a few decades ago, even while doctors were still relying on paternalism to justify their deception of ordinary patients. Instead, "reality orientation" was in vogue, used to force dementia patients to face hard truths, even in the face of tremendous anguish: that a loved one was really dead, for example, or that the patient was now living in a nursing facility and would never go home. But in the 1990s, an Englishwoman named Penny Garner, whose mother, Dorothy, had dementia, began to advocate for a new approach. This was the genesis of validation therapy, which encouraged caregivers to go with the flow of a patient's thoughts, no matter how wrong or deluded or conflicting with reality. "Using the ludicrously simple tactic of agreeing with everything Dorothy said worked like a charm and anything less was disastrous," Garner's son-in-law, Oliver James, wrote about Garner's techniques in his book *Contented Dementia*. Garner told caregivers not to introduce fictions that patients didn't already hold but also not to fight against their comforting delusions either.

In my own career, I have seen how even well-meaning paternalism can be damaging. The doctor-patient relationship is founded on trust, and paternalistic interference not only compromises the relationship but also can erode faith in the profession. For example, studies have shown that patients who have been deceived by their physicians, even if the deception is well intentioned, have reported immense frustration and even thoughts of suicide. Who are we, as doctors, sons, or caregivers, to decide which truths someone can handle?

Truth telling, however, can be a double-edged sword. Its demands may exist in tension with other moral imperatives, such as a son's obligation to do the best for his declining father. Personal ethics, I discovered, may come into conflict with the reality of caregiving.

One Saturday morning about a year after my visit to The Hogeweyk, I woke up to a flurry of texts.

Suneeta: "Dad is kicking Harwinder out again. She is calling her friend and leaving now."

Rajiv: "What happened?"

Suneeta: "He said she doesn't do any work and gets paid $130 a day. She is crying. I'm on the phone with her now."

Rajiv: "I am at a conference. I cannot deal with this right now."

Suneeta: "He is swearing outside and the neighbors are hearing everything. He is saying to let her go and that he doesn't need her. She told me yesterday that if she finds [another job] she is going to leave. She can't work under these conditions anymore. Sandeep, why did you tell him we were paying her??"

Me: "It's his money. If you tell him that she is working for free, he won't believe it or will feel guilty and pay her anyway. Best thing is to tell him the truth. That she is getting paid for the work she is doing."

Rajiv: "You don't understand. He fights with her every time he has to give her a check."

Me: "Then she should leave for a couple days. He will stop when he realizes how much he needs her." (Even as I wrote this, I wasn't sure I believed it.)

Rajiv: "Trust me, that is not the solution. He won't remember. He will do it again."

Me: "If he does it again, she will leave again."

Suneeta: "The poor lady is crying, Sandeep. Sorry, I usually listen to you but not this time. From now on we are going to tell Dad that she is working for free. Rajiv can pay her from Dad's account."

Me: "This gaslighting is bullshit. It confuses him and makes him think that he's going crazy. He knows no one works for free. Just be out with it that she's being paid!"

Rajiv (after a few minutes): "I just spoke to him. He told me he never hired her and never paid her. How do you respond to that?"

Me: "Look, I'm not going to lie to him. He deserves to know what we are doing with his money. If she has to leave, so be it. He's still our father. He understands more than you realize."

Rajiv: "You're wrong. You're still thinking in the old way. He can't even use a cellphone anymore."

Me: "No, you're wrong. He will remember how he feels without her and learn not to misbehave."

Rajiv: "It won't work. He won't remember!"

Me: "And your way has worked perfectly?"

I pulled myself out of bed and walked to the bathroom. I had been on call the previous week, and my head still felt foggy. At the mirror I rubbed the sleep from my eyes. A few minutes later, I heard another ping on my phone.

Rajiv: "I just spoke to Gupta. He told me to increase the Depakote."

We had been taking my father to see Dr. Adarsh Gupta, a psychiatrist friend of Rajiv's, to manage my father's behavior since before my mother died. A jovial man with large white teeth and bushy eyebrows, he'd listened patiently as we narrated my father's most recent temper tantrums or his increasing paranoia. Over the prior two years, he had started my father on daily Lamictal, a mood stabilizer, and Klonopin, an anti-anxiety drug, as needed, both of which we administered. But Lamictal caused a rash all over my father's chest and back, so it was switched to Latuda, which caused my father to smack his lips uncontrollably, a probable sign of a condition called tardive dyskinesia, which is a known side effect (plus it cost $410 a month out of pocket, to boot). Gupta eventually put my father on Lexapro and Wellbutrin for depression and switched Latuda to Depakote for mood stabilization. The latter had to be adjusted downward after my father developed psychomotor slowing, then upward when the rages started up again, with some periods in between when it was stopped altogether. All the while, Gupta prescribed weekly supportive therapy sessions, though I often wondered what the point of therapy was when my father couldn't remember what was discussed from session to session, or even immediately after a session.

Me: "Please, no more Depakote! A blowup every two months is better than him being a zombie."

Rajiv: "Fourth blowup in 4 weeks."

Me: "Depakote makes him angry, too. He was terrible on that visit to Minneapolis. Do not start that medication."

Rajiv: "Gupta says that does not happen. It was only during the bereavement period. He wants us to try it so I am going to. Dad needs mood stabilization."

Me: "He needs to be happy."

Rajiv: "And telling him we're paying Harwinder is going to make him happy?"

I splashed cold water on my face. I applied a dab of toothpaste and started to brush my teeth. I heard the pings of more incoming texts. Squinting at my reflection, I could see my father getting ready for work, clearing his throat, spitting loudly into the sink. I used to feel so sorry for him, for his regimented life, for his failure to relax the constraints that bound him. And now how were things different for any of us?

After I got dressed, I picked up my phone again.

Suneeta: "Dad's like, maybe I made a mistake, everything's fine now. But I could hear Harwinder saying no, I want to leave."

Rajiv: "Suneeta, please call her. Tell her that he doesn't mean it. Sandeep, go over there before she leaves. We can't start this process over again. Please tell him she is working for free. If he asks you if we should pay her, just say no."

Rajiv: "I have no idea anymore what is truth and what is fiction. I can only say that I am exceptionally frustrated and I don't know what to do. He calls me 10 times a day. I pay all his bills and fix his fuckups. His bills have gone to collections 6 times since he moved here for accounts he opened without telling me. I have had to make hours of phone calls on his behalf. I really am at my wit's end. His driver's license expires on his birthday. Now I have to deal with the DMV. Fuck it, I am not going to do it. If he keeps driving, he is going to hurt someone."

Suneeta: "Guys, let's please consider assisted living. I still get emails from Stephanie from that place in Glen Cove. You both should sit down with Dad and convince him."

Rajiv: "I am full board in agreement with assisted living."

Suneeta: "I hate for him to go because I know Dad likes his freedom. But unfortunately, we've tried this for a year and it hasn't worked."

Suneeta (a few minutes later): "Why doesn't Sandeep respond?"

Rajiv: "He probably has us on mute again."

The day was overcast when I left my house. The trees along the Northern State Parkway were leafless and gray. I felt the strange disquietude that autumn always seems to bring, only that year it was more intense than usual. I pictured my car on a wall-sized grid of western Long Island, being pulled by an invisible force toward my father's home, a place I had come to dread, a poisonous node.

Perhaps a nursing home was a foregone conclusion, I thought while driving to Hicksville. In America, one out of six men and women who have dementia live in a nursing facility (more live semi-independently in assisted-living facilities). When Harwinder eventually left, that would surely be the end of my father's independent living. We weren't likely to find another full-time live-in aide, at least not one who cooked Indian food and cared for my father the way Harwinder did. She had been a godsend. Besides housekeeping and preparing meals, she exercised him on the treadmill, walked with him to H&Y Marketplace, and accompanied him to Trader Joe's. Even her friends, when they visited, provided a ready-made social environment. She was doing what his sons had been unable—or unwilling—to do. When she packed up, he would never go willingly to a nursing home or come live with either of us, even if we wanted him to. He would undoubtedly end up in a locked memory unit like his mother. There were no Hogeweyk–style villages on Long Island.

When I pulled into the driveway, the garage door was open. Harwinder came out to meet me. It was obvious she had been crying because there were pink tracks on her tan cheeks. She told me that when my father kicked her out, she had snuck back in through the garage and into the basement, then hid in a closet in the guest room so she could keep an eye on him till I showed up. "He hasn't eaten breakfast," she said. She showed me a bluish discoloration on her skin. "He grabbed my arm. He said, 'I pay you so much. I don't need you.' He called me uneducated, a bitch, a servant. I said, 'I am your servant, but you were a servant to the government. We are all servants on this earth.'"

The storm door was unlocked. When I went inside, my father was sitting at the dining table, staring into his laptop. I greeted him coldly, wanting to make him feel like he had done something wrong. It was my first day off from hospital duty in twelve days, and dealing with another fight he had started with Harwinder over money was the last thing I wanted to be doing that weekend. "Tell me what's going on," I said, sitting down at the table.

"What do you mean, what's going on?"

"You're just sitting here. Did you have lunch?"

He shook his head.

"Then let's eat," I said, nearly shouting. I got up and went to the kitchen. "Where's Harwinder?" I asked. Before he could answer, I said, "I'm sure you lost your temper with her again. That's why she isn't here."

"Don't make assumptions—"

"You did, Dad. I know it."

Harwinder had left rotis wrapped in foil on the counter with some curried cauliflower and okra in Tupperware containers. I heated the leftovers in the microwave and brought them to the table. "Here, you should eat."

My father shook his head. "I am not hungry."

"You're not hungry because you got into a fight with Harwinder."

"Check, maybe she's still here." She had appeared out of thin air so many times after he'd kicked her out that it wasn't hard for him to believe that she would do so again.

"She's not," I barked. "She's gone."

"Okay, I don't care," he said. "I'm fine."

"You're not! Look at yourself. You haven't changed your clothes." He was wearing a white undershirt with curry stains. "At least put on a proper shirt." At that moment, I felt it was necessary to show him how dependent he had become. There was a touch of sadism in this. Memories of all those years he had denigrated me and my common sense and abilities and favored my older brother came rushing forward.

"You're talking to your dad like this? Like he's a stupid man."

"I'm not talking to you like you're a stupid man, but we hired someone to help you and you kicked her out."

"I didn't."

"You did. I know."

"How do you know?"

"She told me everything. You abused her."

"How are you saying I abused her?"

"Screaming at her, pushing her, calling her a bitch, a widow."

"You were there?"

"She has it all on tape." To monitor him remotely, Rajiv had installed a video camera system at the house.

"That's a lie!"

"No, Dad, the tape does not lie. If she's lying, she is the worst woman in the world."

"She is the worst woman."

"Bullshit! Fine, then I'm never going to let her come back. Now that you told me that, we're never going to let her back. I'm not even going to pay her."

"What?"

"She made all this up, right? She's lying, right? So she's not going to get paid."

"She is lying! I swear to God. I swear on anybody's life—"

"Don't! Don't swear on anybody's life. I myself have heard you screaming at her."

"Who?"

"Harwinder!" I shouted, my voice hoarse.

"When?"

"Many times."

"I didn't! I have treated her very well."

"So she's making it all up?"

"People make up things all the time."

"For what reason?"

"To get the upper hand."

The phone rang. He looked at it helplessly. "See, you can't even answer your own phone." I went to pick it up. "Hello." It was Harwinder, still waiting outside. I told her I would call her back.

I came back to the table. Fighting with my ailing father was like allowing your eyes to close momentarily while driving late at night. You know it isn't a good idea. You know your judgment is impaired. But you can't control it.

"Suneeta told me you were upset," I said, softening my tone.

"Sandeep, don't ask me anything. I am the way I am."

"Maybe I can help."

"You can't."

"Maybe talking about it can help."

"I don't want to talk. I have lived my life."

"What does that mean?"

"You should know."

"You're still living, Dad! You're still alive. Take advantage of the time you have, that Mom didn't get. Try to think, what gives you pleasure?"

He thought for a moment. "Work gives me pleasure," he said.

"What gives you pleasure *now*?"

He pounded the table. "Stop it!"

"There are still some things you enjoy, Dad. You like Harwinder. You laugh with her. You like to watch TV. You like to eat. You like to drink juice. You like ice cream, mango lassi; you like all those things. You have to remember what you like." I had hardly finished saying the words before I caught myself. Memory . . .

"You want to talk about Mom?" I said.

"Don't ask me."

"What do you remember about her?" Again, I caught myself.

"Everything. She was a nice lady."

"What's your favorite"—I couldn't think of a better word—"memory?"

"She helped me a lot."

"She was supportive?"

"Very supportive."

"How did she help you?"

He struggled to remember. "Everything," he finally said, motioning for me to stop talking. He must have felt sorry for me because he added, "Don't worry about anything."

"I'm not worried, Dad. You're just going to be alone here."

"I'll be alone," he said resignedly. "It's okay. Don't worry."

When he was done eating, I took him upstairs for his nap. I helped him take off his shirt and put on a clean one. He lay down on the bed, and I pulled the comforter over him. "Put your head up," I said as I pushed a hard pillow under him so he could watch TV. I sat down on a chair near his bedside. We stayed in silence for a few minutes.

"Rajiv and Suneeta say that if this lady leaves . . ."

"Which lady?"

"Harwinder. If she leaves, we are going to have to put you in a nursing home. I am the only one who's stopping them from doing it. Do you think I want you to go to a nursing home?"

"Don't tell me what you want or what I want," he said bitterly.

"You can't take care of yourself, Dad."

"Okay, let me die then. Let me go to hell!"

I stood up. "You know, you're not the only one who ever lost a spouse," I said. I mentioned one of my patients with heart failure. She lived alone. Her sons visited her maybe once a week. She couldn't afford a housekeeper like Harwinder. She had to do the cooking and shopping herself. And yet she was happy every time she came to see me. "Happiness is a state of mind," I said. At this, he looked up and nodded. This he seemed to understand. He had been saying it himself for years.

I went downstairs to the kitchen. Harwinder was creeping up the basement steps. Without saying a word, I motioned for her to follow me. We walked up to the bedroom.

She was standing behind me when my father opened his eyes. "Look, Dad, Harwinder came back," I said. He eyed her suspiciously. "She says she is sorry. She told me she will work for free. No money. Just food and shelter."

His face relaxed, and I discerned a faint smile. "Okay," he said. "Please come in."

10

WELL, DON'T WORRY ABOUT MY LONELINESS!

Unfortunately, the fights didn't end that day. They got worse as my father's disability grew and Harwinder, by her very presence, reminded him of his helplessness and decline. I'd watch him on the surveillance system my brother had set up at the house. Much of the time he got along well with Harwinder, but sometimes he behaved abominably—calling her a two-bit whore, throwing orange juice at her face, even on one occasion grabbing her by the throat and then, a few minutes later, bending down on his knees, touching her feet, begging for forgiveness as she angrily ignored him. "In a nursing home, they would give him an injection," she told me bitterly after he tried to hit her with a wire hanger. "Here, I am giving him tea and snacks."

Of course, my siblings and I felt a responsibility to stop such abuse. We spoke to my father about it constantly, cajoling, shouting, even threatening to put him in an institution. Still, we could not get him to understand or control his outbursts. So, not knowing what else to do, we talked with Harwinder about how we could make it right. She eventually agreed to weekly bonuses as a form of hazard pay. In addition, my sister bought her gifts, and we sent money to her children. She had an extraordinary devotion to our family, especially to

Suneeta, with whom she had a genuine friendship, and we felt the need to reward her for her loyalty and to compensate her for her hardships. At the same time, we were desperate. Her live-in caregiving allowed us to function at our careers and in our families. Plus, it was the only thing keeping my father out of a nursing home.

My father's life, on video, was in fact like a series of video loops. There he was again, walking to the front door, looking out onto the porch, then coming back to his chair at the dining table to stare again at the TV. At other times he would wander through the garage, poking at various things, occasionally picking up old newspapers, pretending to read them. These sequences would be repeated throughout the day. I witnessed it all from my office at work. Both father and son had developed a tolerance for tedium.

When I'd play the tapes of him shouting at her, he would look resigned. "Is that you?" I'd ask disappointedly. "Yes, probably," he'd admit. But when I would mention the abuse even a minute later, he'd cry, "What! I never abused her."

"I just played you the tape!"

"Show me," he'd insist, and we would go through it all over again. Our conversations were like a carousel, revisiting the same point again and again at regularly spaced intervals. As a physician I knew the futility of what I was doing. Yet as a son I continued to hold out some hope for understanding.

Still, he would deny his bad behavior every time. No matter how hard I tried to kindle in him a flicker of insight into what he had done, he would remain impassive, aloof, indifferent, unconcerned. "'Whore' is not a dirty word," he'd explain to me as Harwinder wept in her room. "It is just something you say."

At times I thought that he was putting me on, that his lack of self-awareness was self-serving. Perhaps it was a manifestation of his fragile ego, his unwillingness to admit mistakes, his historical disdain for introspection, or maybe the optimism he'd always credited himself with. It wasn't until a visit to St. Louis later that fall that I began to recognize it as mostly a consequence of his brain disease.

In St. Louis, I met Dr. Gregory Day, a young neurologist at the Washington University School of Medicine. Trim and talkative, Day was the associate head of research at the Charles F. and Joanne Knight Alzheimer's Disease Research Center, a complex of red brick buildings just off the main campus where I'd gone to medical school. We spoke in his office on a chilly November morning; frost speckled the patch of grass outside his window. I started our conversation by asking Day about my father's seeming lack of self-awareness. Even more than his memory trouble, it was his inability to monitor or regulate how he was thinking and behaving that was creating an intolerable strain at home.

Day told me that loss of insight into one's own impeded functioning, or *anosognosia*, is common in several neurological conditions, including dementia. "It's one of the challenges but also one of the fascinating things working in brain disorders," he said. "Neurology involves a consciousness but also a metaconsciousness that we don't necessarily see in other diseases." The term "anosognosia" was coined about a century ago to describe stroke patients who seemed unaware of their paralysis. Though the phenomenon remains poorly understood, it is observed today in a host of neurological and psychiatric conditions—including traumatic brain injury, obsessive-compulsive disorder, and schizophrenia—in which awareness of the disease and its consequences is compromised by the disease itself. Anosognosia can vary in severity, from mild to profound, and in the exact mental domain affected. A person might be aware of decline in one area of functioning, such as memory, but not in another, such as empathy or sociability. For example, a person with frontotemporal dementia, a relatively rare form of the disease, might not know that picking your nose in public or rubbing the back of someone you've never met is inappropriate but still might recognize that their memories are failing.

I wondered if anosognosia is a form of amnesia. Perhaps my father was relying on distant memories of a distant self—when he was intact, mild-tempered, a family man, a scientist—memories that hadn't disappeared despite the slow destruction of his brain. Day sees it differently. He believes anosognosia is a structural problem with a specific neurological substrate. "Parts of the brain obviously perform meta [or higher order] functions," he told me. One of those activities is self-awareness, he added, which is controlled by networks in the frontal and parietal lobes that are involved in both self-monitoring and the motivation to correct error. Individuals like my father who have suffered damage to these areas often lack insight into their deficits—including the fact that they no longer have such insight.

It is a sad dynamic: being unaware of, or unable to think about, one's disease because of the disease. I'd seen it in medical school on the neurology wards. Patients with a parietal stroke might not be able to move the limbs on the left side of their body, but you wouldn't know it from asking them. They would deny that there was anything wrong with them and, when faced with evidence of their disability, would confabulate reasons why their limbs were not functioning. They didn't seem to care that they were grievously impaired. They thought their deficit was your problem, not theirs.

I asked Day why my mother had retained insight into her condition. For example, she knew till the very end that her visual hallucinations were not real, even as she was having them. Parkinson's disease, Day explained, has a very different pathology from Alzheimer's, and this may account for the difference in the degree of self-awareness. Parkinson's usually starts in the motor-control part of the brain called the basal ganglia and then moves out to cortical areas. "Depending on where it goes, that sort of defines the syndromes that people have," he said. Damage to the limbic system results in behavioral changes, such as irrational behaviors. Disease in the brain stem causes fluctuations in consciousness, fainting spells, and so on. If the damage extends to the occipital lobe, there are hallucinations and visual problems. However, in my mother's brain, the frontal and parietal lobes were probably spared. Therefore, despite her encroaching disabilities, she was still able to step outside of them to assess them.

Alzheimer's disease, on the other hand, often causes damage to the frontal and parietal lobes, though usually only in the latter stages. At an early stage of the disease, patients may retain insight and actually complain or make jokes about their failing memories, like Henry Molaison did. They may be even more aware of their deficits than their family members. However, by the time the disease reaches its middle stages, usually two to five years after diagnosis, insight and self-awareness frequently have begun to deteriorate. Patients may still know they have a memory problem, for example, but they have forgotten the extent of it. This was likely how the disease had played out in my father's brain. He had insight early on into the changes that were unfolding in him. He decided to retire, after all, and move to Long Island to live near his sons. He knew something was wrong, even if he was apt to deny it more and more as his disease progressed. But by the time I made my trip to St. Louis in the fall of 2017, his self-awareness was disintegrating; he was confined to the corrupted reality that his brain had created.

Day acknowledged that there is so much plasticity in the brain that we can't say for sure where the regions controlling some functions lie. On average, certain functions, such as insight, map to certain regions, but there is substantial variability. Some patients with advanced dementia, for example, retain significant insight. Others with relatively early disease may have a total lack of it. "The structure-function imbalance is something we live with on a regular basis," he said. "We may see people with normal functioning on cognitive testing, and then you image their brain, and they have a shriveled walnut sitting up there."

He suggested I watch a video his department used to train its neurology fellows. In the video, a seventy-four-year-old retired manager for Southwestern Bell came to the clinic with his wife of thirty-one years.* "We didn't recognize [the problem] right away," the woman told the doctor about her husband's memory trouble. "Then he'd ask me five times what day it was."

The man's story had a familiar ring. There was his growing inability to cope with small sums of money or follow driving directions or operate the TV remote. He had suffered a loss of social relationships, too. He'd dropped out of his bridge club. He stopped going to the YMCA after he put his belongings into the wrong locker and couldn't find them. There were problems with judgment, too. He'd tried to mow the lawn when the grass was wet, gumming up the mower blades. But in at least one respect his disease was less advanced than my father's. "I forget things that I shouldn't," he admitted with appropriate insight as his wife looked on sadly.

Before leaving that day, I asked Day if there was anything new or on the horizon that could help my father. He said nothing for a few moments. Then he replied, "I'm sure you're aware that none of our disease-modifying medications work one bit in people who already have symptoms. If we wait till people have dementia, the freight train has left the station and we can't slow it down. Anyone who says they can is lying or trying to make money off of you."

I felt strangely relieved to hear this. I'd been feeling guilty for not looking harder for novel or experimental therapies, but Day's comment was a reminder that no such effective treatments existed. I thanked him for his time and got up to leave.

"Does your father still know you?" he asked.

"Yes," I said.

* For clinical assessments, patients are required to come in with caregivers who can provide their own history. The discrepancy between how caregivers and patients rate a problem is used to measure patients' insight.

"Calls you by name?"

"Most of the time." Sometimes he would forget the names of his grandchildren, I told him, but he still knew who I was and was usually happy to see me.

He asked where my father was living. I said that he was still in his own home with a full-time aide and that we were trying to keep him out of an institutional setting for as long as possible.

"It sounds like you are doing everything you can to ensure his safety and preserve his quality of life," Day said sympathetically. "Now it's just a matter of resources—paid caregivers, for example."

He paused as if trying to think of something else to offer.

Then he said sadly: "But unfortunately, in the end, all dementias look alike. The whole brain is affected. Patients generally can't speak."

The conundrum we faced after my mother died was how to convince an already stubborn man—and now one without insight into his own condition and needs—to accept additional help. On Sundays, Harwinder's day off, my father would go out by himself and get lost. He would turn on the stove to make tea and forget to turn it off. He would skip meals because he couldn't heat up the food that Harwinder had prepared since he'd forgotten how to use the microwave. Rajiv and I staggered our weekend hospital schedules so one of us would always be available to assist him, but it was a stop-gap solution because neither of us could be with him every moment of the day.

We were relieved when my aunt Krishna, my father's youngest and only living sibling, visited from India the following summer. My father had invited her to stay with him before my mother died over two years earlier, but by the time she arrived, he wanted nothing to do with her. A widow herself, she wanted to talk, share, support him in his time of need, but he found it impossible to disguise his distaste for her presence.

"She is your family," we told him.

"She is not my family."

"She is your sister."

"So what!"

Before a week had passed, he had had enough. "I'll be so happy when you leave," he told her, causing her to pack her bags. She spent much of the remainder of her time in America with a distant cousin in New Jersey.

So my father was alone as usual when I pulled up to his house one Sunday in October 2018 to take him to lunch. On the lawn, yellow leaves had collected, and the summer plantings were scarred and already beginning to wilt. I found him sitting on his bed, struggling to get dressed. It had been taking him longer to put on his clothes, especially if it was cold outside and he needed to wear layers. Sometimes he would put his shoes on before his pants, or a sweater on before a shirt, or a sweater on top of another sweater. Frequently he would forget to start with underwear.

I walked over to help him. "Let's put your shirt on," I said, trying to get him to stand up. The garment was pulled inside out, so I quickly reversed it, then offered him a hole for his arm. "Wait, that's not right," I said, pulling it off. "Can you stand up?"

"What are you doing?" he thundered.

"You put the shirt on backwards. Stand up and move over here."

"Sandeep, don't tell me one hundred things: 'Stand up, move here, go there.'"

"I am trying to help you. Do you want me to help you or not?"

"No," he barked.

"Fine, do it yourself." I turned and defiantly walked out of the room, before whirling around in the knowledge that otherwise I'd be waiting for God-knows-how-long downstairs. "Please, Dad," I said. "Can we just get this done?"

After he was done getting dressed, we had another time-consuming task to perform: leaving the house. First, we looked for his keys. They were under some papers on the dining table. Then we went around the house flipping the lights off (before he made another pass to flip some of them back on). He stepped onto the porch to check the mailbox. (It was Sunday.) Then he went back inside, leaving me standing on the front steps.

"Where are you going?"

"I don't know where I put my keys."

"You just checked them," I shouted, but he was already gone.

When I found him upstairs, he was applying Scotch tape to his closet door, presumably to keep it from being opened in his absence.

"What are you doing?" I cried, beginning to lose my temper.

"Okay, let's go," he said quickly, leaving the roll of tape dangling.

"Did you find your keys?"

"Yes."

"Where were they?" I asked as we walked out of the bedroom.

"In my pocket," he said.

Outside, the sun was shining, though the temperature wasn't much above fifty degrees. Wind chimes sounded in the light breeze. An American flag flapped on a pole in the distance.

In the car, I latched his seatbelt before backing out of the driveway. "So, where should we go?" I asked brightly, trying to infuse some excitement into our weekly ritual.

"Don't ask me," he replied flatly.

The neighborhood around our usual place, House of Dosas, was dotted with South Asian establishments. We drove past a Bengali sweets shop, a halal butchery, and a sari boutique before parking in the crowded lot. Weeds were growing through cracks in the blacktop. Cold steam was rising from the gutters.

"I've been here before, I think," my father said. "Is this Diwan Grill?"

"No, it's House of Dosas. We come here every week."

"Every week?" he said incredulously.

"Yes, Dad, we've been here every Sunday for the past six weeks."

I opened the car door for him, and he gingerly set his feet down on the asphalt. He had on his usual get-up: olive green slacks, dark brown leather jacket, and shiny black leather shoes. The pajamas he'd insisted on wearing were visible under the fraying cuffs of his trousers. There was a bulge under his sweater from the wallet and other crap he'd stuffed into his shirt pocket. He bent his knees but did not move. I offered my hand. "I have become old," he said. Then, for the first time in what seemed like weeks, he laughed.

We held hands crossing the parking lot. At the Diwali celebration going on across the street, families were waiting in a makeshift line for grilled corn and spicy chaat. Teens with orange scarves on their heads were standing next to their parents as I once had, hands in pockets, just waiting to go home.

The restaurant had low wooden beams and tinted windows and was dark and cool, like a church. Wooden carvings of Hindu deities graced the walls. When the proprietor saw us in the waiting area, we were hurriedly seated.

"Where is that lady?" my father asked after we sat down.

"Who? Harwinder? She doesn't work on Sunday, remember?"

"Why not?"

"Because you said you didn't want her."

His eyes narrowed as he thought about what I'd said. Then he nodded, obviously pleased that he retained some say in such matters.

"What kind of dosa do you want?" I asked.

"You decide," he replied. So when the waitress came over, I ordered two spicy dosas with semolina crust, his favorite. This was happening more and more. Dementia was shutting down his ability to identify what he wanted, or even feel that he wanted it. Increasingly, the onus was on me to remember for him.

We sat quietly. I could see that his fingernails were getting long, so I made a mental note to clip them when we got home. I also noticed that his Seiko wristwatch had stopped. He was wearing it simply as an adornment.

"Sandeep, what is this thing?" he said. On his flip phone he showed me an invitation he had received to join the editorial board of an agricultural science journal. I looked over the email. I was surprised anyone had thought to reach out to him—he had been retired for more than four years.

"Do you know this journal?" I asked.

"Yes," he said, but I could tell he was lying.

"'You have done great work in the field of plant biotechnology,'" I read out loud. He looked on with pride. "'Therefore, we would like to invite you to review—'"

"How do I tell them I don't want to do it?" he said, interrupting me.

I searched his face for some sign of regret, but it remained expressionless. "Are you sure?" I asked.

"Yes," he replied. So, sad but relieved, I painstakingly instructed him on how to type out a declination.

The waitress brought over two triangular dosas filled with curried potato, two bowls of spicy sambar soup, and two glasses of mango lassi. My father asked her for a pipe. I quickly passed him a plastic straw.

"Do you ever miss India?" I said as we settled into our meals.

"What do you mean?"

"Do you ever miss India?" I repeated.

"The show?"

I had no idea what he meant by this. "No, the country."

"Oh, India is hell," he said dismissively. "I have not been to India in twenty years." In fact, he had gone to India for a month only six years earlier, to deliver a series of invited lectures, "From Green Revolution to Gene Revolution," at major universities.

"What's wrong with India?"

"Well"—he hesitated—"whenever you have partition and so on."

"The partition was well before, Dad. I'm talking about when we lived there before coming to America."

"When was the partition?"

"1947. I'm talking about when we lived there in 1975."

He shrugged his shoulders and continued to pick at his meal.

It was the sort of apathetic response I had come to expect from him. Once a perfectionist, he no longer seemed to care about making mistakes, or why he'd made them, or even to register that he was impaired. By then I understood that it was beyond his control—my conversation the previous fall with Dr. Day in St. Louis had convinced me of this—but I still couldn't resist the urge to correct him when he erred, to embarrass him a little, to remind him, a man of science, that errors were still important.

At the same time, I recognized the benefits of his obliviousness. The man who'd craved recognition and respect from others more than anything else no longer seemed to care about those fickle rewards. His brain was shrinking, no doubt, but so too were his imaginings, perceptions, ambitions, and expectations—and maybe that was not such a bad thing. I sometimes thought of the oncologist with metastatic pancreatic cancer whom I'd once treated as a resident at Memorial Sloan Kettering: the knowledge of what was surely to come corroded the little time the man had left. This was something we didn't have to worry about with my father. His loss of insight was actually a protective mechanism. In a way, the illness was taking care of itself.

There were other consolations, too. We could lie about things that never happened in order to assuage his anxiety (I had long since gotten over my taboo of lying to him)—for instance, telling him, "Rajiv called you before he left for his trip," when in fact he did not. More-over, the things that used to upset him no longer did. He would forget arguments quickly. He didn't fixate on the denials or the rebukes. With little short-term memory, he was passing through life in a kind of hallucinatory state. Within minutes, sometimes less, his mood could change from rage to resignation to something that approximated joy, or at least mischief or playfulness—a playfulness he had never had when I was growing up. I would stew over our arguments only to call and hear him cry, "Hello, young man!" He was living in the pure present, even if it was just an artifact of his disease. His ability to forget was a blessing as well as a curse.

"How is your dosa?" He was still working on one vertex of the folded triangle. The whole thing was clearly going to be too much for him.

"Fine," he said, without looking up. "It's good."

"Here, let me put some sauce on it." He loved—or used to love—coconut chutney. But he waved me off; he wasn't going to eat much more.

Sitting with him, I remembered our lunches during my first year as an undergraduate at Berkeley, when he was working temporarily as a postdoc at a plant genetics research center a few miles away in Albany, California. Every Sunday he would bring me to his apartment, where he would have spent the morning preparing curried chicken livers with homemade yogurt—my favorite—and deliver a stern lecture about what I should do with my life. He'd always wanted me to become a doctor—one trained at Stanford, no less. To him, that was the apogee of professional attainment. I wanted nothing to do with his dream. (In immigrant Indian culture, youthful rebellion is saying no to a career in medicine—but then majoring, as I did, in experimental physics.) Still, he continued to push. He always believed that a loved one could be worked on, persuaded, set on the right track—that one more admonishment or warning from him could avert disaster.

Now, more than thirty years later, our roles reversed, I was kind of hoping that was true.

"It must be hard for you to be alone on Sundays," I said, by way of starting another conversation about getting more help from Harwinder. "Why don't you visit Suneeta for a few days?"

He eyed me suspiciously. "Very good idea," he said sarcastically.

I felt my temperature rise. "Why is it not a good idea? The house is quiet now that Krishna is gone. So I am offering you an option."

"That's the worst option."

"Why is it not a good option?"

"Well, you have to go there, go to the airport," he said vaguely.

"It's not that hard, Dad. Rajiv will drop you off on the plane. It lands in Minneapolis, and Suneeta will pick you up. It's not that complicated."

"Then come back and go through the same miserable time. What will Suneeta do? No," he said, shaking his head. "I am fine."

He'd been a lifelong traveler. I still remember the elaborate slideshows of his trips to European conferences he used to show us: the Tower of London, the fountains of Brussels. Now he wouldn't fly even three hours to Minneapolis.

"You're not fine," I said, trying to resist the urge to slide into another full-blown argument. "You told Suneeta this morning that you are lonely."

"I told her that?"

"Yes."

"Well, don't worry about my loneliness!"

"I am just trying to help you."

"You are not trying to help."

"So I am trying to hurt then? That's what you think? I was the one who set up the Cold Spring Harbor tour for you, remember? I set up the Hofstra scholarship. I took you to that luncheon."

"Which luncheon?"

"The luncheon at Hofstra when you got the plaque. We walked up there, remember? It's so easy to criticize."

"That's what you are doing."

"Look, all I'm saying is, you can visit Suneeta, or . . . I don't know . . . maybe we can have Harwinder stay at the house on Sundays, too."

He fixed his eyes on me. "Harwinder doesn't have her own family?"

This provided an opening. "Harwinder told Suneeta that she wants to stay with you seven days a week now, just as long as she gets a couple of days off a month."

He started to shake his head.

"Why not, Dad? You're happier when she's at the house, right? She serves you well—and she needs a place to stay. It helps her, it helps you."

"She pushed me, remember?" he said as the memory of her holding him back from striking her during one of their rows surfaced.

"Mm-hmm. What for?"

"I don't know."

"Did you do something? You remember the push. What about what you did?"

"I did nothing."

"I see, so she's so crazy that she'll push you for no reason," I said, realizing the conversation was devolving like all the others had. "You must have done something, Dad. You only remember the things that suit you!"

He insisted on paying the bill, as he always did, but I told him he could pay next time, as I always did. He did not believe in tipping. Like many Indians of his generation, he viewed it as an affectation, to be proffered only for good service, never automatically, and rarely at more than 5 percent. So, rather than deal with the disappointed stares from the waitstaff, I paid the bill.

"I like this place," my father said as we walked out. "We should come every week."

Back in the car, I put on Nusrat Fateh Ali Khan. The qawwali began with a sitar riff before the tabla drums took over and Khan began to belt out his lyrics. My father, once an avid listener of Sufi Muslim poetry, quietly snapped his fingers to the tune.

Glad to see him a bit relaxed, I took a detour on the way home and drove ten miles to the bay near Centre Island. We had gone there once before when my mother was alive, and I remembered my father had enjoyed the walk along the dunes. After parking along the road, we hopped over a short wooden fence and walked onto the beach. It was overcast by then, the gray clouds coalescing into big lumps in the sky. Yellow tangles of dry grass stood up in the white sand. Off in the distance, the Long Island Sound shimmered like a pool of mercury. A few bickering seagulls flew overhead, but otherwise the place was deathly quiet.

"What are we doing here?" my father said.

I reached out for his hand. "We're just walking," I replied.

Near the shore, the air was even cooler. Seaweed in varying stages of decay lay along the bank. Tiny waves percolated into a reddish froth in the sand.

"Remember when we used to walk on the beach in Aberystwyth?"

"Where?"

"Aberystwyth, Wales. Remember? There was a boardwalk. I was five years old."

"Yes, I remember. It was a four-bedroom house. Suneeta was born there."

"And Mom worked as a seamstress."

He nodded. He was staring out beyond the bay to Connecticut. "She was a great woman," he said. "She went very fast."

"But that is the best way to go, don't you think? How would you want to go when it is your time?"

He put up his hand. "Let's not talk, please," he said.

We came to a pool of water surrounded by green grass. Minute ripples were traveling across the surface, disappearing at the edges like lines of static. We stood at the edge. "What are we doing here, Sandeep?" he asked again.

I knew the end was coming. All these moments together—the lunches and walks, the memories he'd neglected to transfer before it was too late, stories of when I was too young to form and retain my own memories—were going to be lost, like the ripples on a pond.

There was nothing left to do now but walk. Walk together, side by side, till the end. What lay ahead of us, I couldn't say. Would he forget me? How much would I forget him? How long would he be able to process that this was a beach, and his relationship to it? When would those black-and-white letters cease to be a sign?

"You used to drive a scooter in India," I said as we stared into the pool.

"What?"

"You used to drive me on your scooter. To the Pusa Institute. That is where your lab was, remember? We lived in Kirti Nagar. Mataji used to live with us."

"Where?"

"In Kirti Nagar. Mom used to teach at the high school. Rajiv and I went to Delhi Public School. The teachers used to slap us when we gave the wrong answer. Remember?"

"I remember," he said.

"You used to bring me balloons. You tied them to the back of the scooter. When you got home, I used to release them—"

He put up his hand. "Let's go back," he interrupted, getting antsy. "I am tired."

"You don't want to walk some more?"

"No," he said. "Let's go home." I could tell he was exhausted and would not be dissuaded. So we turned and headed back.

"I am glad you came," he said as we retraced our footsteps in the damp sand.

I glanced over at him, surprised by the sentiment. "Me too, Dad."

"It has been many days since I've seen you, I think."

"I saw you yesterday."

He started to laugh. "Sorry, I forgot." We took a few steps. "Sanja, we always liked you," he said.

Now it was my turn to laugh. "Who's 'we'?"

"Me, my wife. You were always bright. You were at the top."

"So were you, Dad. They used to call you Topper."

"No," he cried. "Topmost."

"I think Topper, Dad."

He shrugged. "Might be. I am glad we came."

"Me too," I said.

"We should do this more often. I learn things from you."

"Like what?"

"Like be more pleasant. Don't sulk."

"Well, we'll do it again next week. Harwinder will be back in the morning."

"Next time, bring Pia."

"I will."

"Will you remember?"

"I'll remember."

"You are very forgetful. What did I tell you?"

"'Bring Pia.'"

He laughed. "Your memory is good." He stopped suddenly. "Let's go back. I'm tired."

"The car is up ahead, Dad, on the road. We have to keep walking."

"It has been a long journey," my father said.

"I know," I said as we started to walk again. "But it's almost over."

11

WHERE IS YOUR MOM?

Who am I? This or the other?
Am I one person today and tomorrow another?

—DIETRICH BONHOEFFER, German theologian

What does it mean to be a person? The eighteenth-century Enlightenment philosopher David Hume theorized that a person is simply a collection of experiences written into the code of memory. In his *Treatise of Human Nature*, he wrote, "When I enter most intimately into what I call myself, I always stumble on some particular perception or other." He went on to say that a person is "nothing but a bundle or collection of different perceptions, which succeed each other with an inconceivable rapidity, and are in a perpetual flux and movement." These impressions and perceptions are fleeting, he asserted. Memory lends them a sense of continuity and connectedness, so they are boxed together into episodes of experience. "Had we no memory," he wrote, "we never should have any notion of causation, nor consequently of that chain of causes and effects, which constitute our self or person."

Therefore, in Hume's conception, our personal identities are tied to what we can remember. Once you lose your memories, have you not also lost your "self?"

In *An Essay Concerning Human Understanding*, John Locke, the Enlightenment philosopher, similarly wrote that the hallmark of personhood is a personal consciousness that identifies itself with its previous actions and experiences. A person, he wrote, is a "thinking intelligent being, that has reason and reflection, and can consider itself as itself, the same thinking thing in different times and places." In this cognitive-centric view, the self is undergirded by memory. Without memory, we would float away into oblivion like a boat untied from its pier. To Locke, it was the conscious self that constituted the person. He wrote, "As far as consciousness can be extended backwards to any past action or thought, so far reaches the identity of that person." In other words, a person's identity is maintained by the memories that link his former state with his present one.

A modern interpretation of this idea was put forward by the contemporary philosopher Derek Parfit, who defined a person as bundles of connected memories, intentions, thoughts, and desires. Parfit discussed a thought experiment in which a person's body and brain are scanned down to their exact cellular state, and the information is beamed to Mars, where it is used to create a replica of the original person. This replica, with its identical brain and body, looks, thinks, behaves, and remembers past experiences exactly like the original person. If the person is now sacrificed, is it not reasonable to say that he lives on in the replica?

Parfit's view, embodied in the Western values of autonomy and rationality, is a cognitive-centric perspective. It defines a person as the continuous bridging of thoughts, perceptions, and desires—in other words, mental states—over time. From this perspective, your personhood is just the movie that has been running over your lifetime, stretching back into the past (at least back to your preschool years, when long-term memory begins) and projecting into the future. In the absence of psychological continuity—embodied in memory—personal identity loses its meaning. In a sense, nursing homes like The Hogeweyk are trying to restore psychological continuity through physical links to, and reminders of, a past life.

However, when you define a human being only by his mental life, there is a slippery slope leading to dehumanization. For example, Parfit wrote that "a person can gradually cease to exist some time before his heart stops beating." He added, "We can plausibly claim that if the person has ceased to exist, we have no moral reason to help his heart go on beating, or to refrain from preventing this."

Other modern thinkers have advanced similar views about people living with severe dementia. For instance, Peter Singer, the Princeton ethicist, has written that the euthanasia of neurologically devastated infants or adults with advanced dementia is no great moral transgression. "Only a person can want to go on living, or have plans for the future, because only a person can even understand the possibility of a future existence for herself or himself," Singer wrote in his 1994 book *Rethinking Life and Death*. He went on: "This means that to end the lives of people, against their will, is different from ending the lives of beings who are not people. Indeed, strictly speaking, in the case of those who are not people, we cannot talk of ending their lives against or in accordance with their will, because they are not capable of having a will on such a matter." In another book, *Practical Ethics*, Singer wrote, "That a being is a human being . . . is not relevant to the wrongness of killing it. It is rather characteristics like rationality, autonomy, and self-consciousness that make a difference."

These philosophical beliefs have even received legal sanction. In March 2003, Kenneth Edge, a seventy-nine-year-old Scottish man who'd smothered with a pillow his demented eighty-five-year-old wife, Winifred, to whom he had been married for fifty-five years, received no punishment or fine other than a verbal warning. The judge in the case, Lady Smith, took note of "the enormous stresses and strains you had been put under as you tried to care for a woman who ceased to be the woman you married."

However, to paraphrase the neonatologist John Wyatt, how can the integrity of a few collections of neurons in the hippocampus (and perhaps also in the cortex and thalamus) determine whether a human being has personhood and is therefore entitled to the rights, moral protections, and respect that such a designation entails? How can a monumental characteristic such as personhood boil down to just a few brain parts?

There is a competing philosophical perspective. It holds that the psychological "continuity" believed to underlie personhood is never continuous anyway. For example, I may not remember an experience I had as a child, but I do remember being a young adult, and when I was a young adult, I did remember the experience I had as a child. Therefore, if the present me is the same person as the young adult, and the young adult is the same person as the child, then, even in the absence of psychological continuity, I must still be the same person as the child. So obviously memory alone cannot fully determine personal identity.

Moreover, in this perspective, psychological continuity is not served by memory alone. It is also served by intentions, beliefs, values, habits, and other unconscious behaviors that are often preserved in patients with severe dementia.

Even the claim that psychological continuity is essential for personhood has its flaws. A person is contained in a system of other people. We are not just our intellects but also our relationships, our connections, and our interactions; these things also give our lives meaning and contribute to personhood. For example, my father may not have remembered that we went to House of Dosas for lunch every Sunday, but he still knew that I was the person who took him there, wherever it was. We still shared a family relationship and a shared history, even if he didn't always remember the relationship or the history himself. He was still my father because I thought of him as such.

The social psychologist Tom Kitwood has argued that reducing the self to cognitive competency is a flawed—and essentially academic—exercise. He wrote, "Behind such debates a vague shadow can be discerned. It is that of the liberal academic of former times: kind, considerate, honest, fair, and above all else intellectual. Emotion and feeling have only a minor part in this scheme of things; autonomy is given supremacy over relationship and commitment; passion has no place at all."

In other words, the conventional paradigm about what constitutes a person does not give adequate import to the richness of a human being outside of his cognitive capacities. Human beings exist not only in an inner world but also in a public space. It is that space that continues to give meaning to the lives of people living with severe dementia. As the twentieth-century theologian Martin Buber put it: "Spirit is not in the I, but between I and Thou. It is not like the blood that circulates in you, but like the air in which you breathe."

In the winter, I took my father back to see Dr. Gordon. Four years had elapsed since our first visit, and my father's condition had clearly worsened. His mini-mental exam score was now 17 out of 30—previously it was about 24—a clear progression into moderate dementia. It was hard to know how much of the decline was because of depression following my mother's death, but my father's psychological state notwithstanding, his brain disease had clearly progressed. An MRI scan now showed "worsening microvascular ischemic changes in the white matter," suggesting "vascular" dementia caused by blockages in the brain's blood vessels (perhaps stemming from my father's longstanding and poorly treated high blood pressure). But there was also "midbrain volume loss" and "disproportionate temporal lobe volume loss in the region of the hippocampus," suggesting Alzheimer's as well. The complexity of my father's behavior, the maddening incomprehensibility of it, was right there on the scan, boiled down to a few millimeter-sized changes in his scarring brain.

Vascular abnormalities in the brain, Gordon told us, often coexist with plaques and tangles. In fact, mixed-type dementia is now believed to be the most common form in older patients, though the designation remains essentially academic because no good treatments are available for either type.* Nevertheless, there are measures people can take to lower the risk of developing dementia in the first place: eating a healthy diet, for example, and getting enough exercise. In 2015 a Finnish study showed that following a Mediterranean-type diet rich in whole grains, fish, and fruits and vegetables improved cognitive performance and decision-making among older adults over a two-year span. Similar studies have shown that higher levels of physical activity—even simple housework like cooking and cleaning—are associated with better cognition in older adults, even when brain lesions, such as amyloid plaques, are present.

Other measures that have shown preventive benefit include getting enough sleep, engaging in social and cognitive activities that stimulate the brain, avoiding smoking and heavy drinking, and minimizing stress. Many of these measures minimize cardiovascular risk, too. In fact, there is strong evidence today that cardiovascular risk factors are also risk factors for dementia. A modeling study has es-

---

* For much of the twentieth century, vascular dementia was believed to be the main cause of brain degeneration in the elderly. Then the pendulum swung to Alzheimer's disease. Today, however, the importance of vascular lesions in Alzheimer's is increasingly being recognized. Multiple pathologies, it is now believed, may combine to create the degenerative brain state typical of the disease.

timated that even modest reductions in cardiovascular risk factors like diabetes, hypertension, obesity, smoking, and physical inactivity could reduce the total number of Alzheimer's cases by 1 million worldwide.

Though the MRI didn't explain it, my father's gait had also become unstable. That winter was the winter of the falls. One night after Christmas 2018, he fell in his bedroom on the way to the bathroom, hitting his head on the wooden floor. We immediately stopped his aspirin (a blood thinner), as well as the Alzheimer's drug Exelon, which Dr. Gordon had started, but the tumbles continued. He fell again two weeks later after inexplicably going on his treadmill in the dark. "I made a mistake," he admitted disconsolately when I shouted at him, asking why he had taken such a stupid risk, but I knew it was only a matter of time before a major fall.

It happened one sunny evening in the spring of 2019. We got a call from Harwinder that my father had taken a terrible spill just up the street from his house. He'd tripped again on a crack in the sidewalk, this time faceplanting on the concrete and opening a gash just above his right eye. He had passed out for a few seconds.

I met my brother and father in the parking lot at Walgreen's, where Rajiv had driven them to buy bandages and supplies to clean my father's wounds. Reclining in the back seat, my father appeared dazed. Blood was dripping from the wound above his eye and from the hand he had used to break his fall. However, he denied he was in any pain and said he just wanted to go to bed. We knew it would be a long night if we took him to the emergency room, even if we pulled rank with our hospital privileges, so after getting the supplies we needed, we took him home.

He fell out of bed twice that night. I was supposed to fly out to London for a book award ceremony the following morning. I thought about cancelling the trip, but Rajiv insisted that I go. Just before boarding the plane, I got a call from him from the North Shore University

Hospital emergency department, where he'd taken my father to be evaluated. A CT scan had just revealed that my father had a subdural hematoma, a collection of blood just under the skull, with bleeding extending into the brain. It was still a relatively small bleed, but doctors had decided to admit him to the hospital for observation.

He stayed in the hospital for three days. It was a difficult time, as my brother relayed in daily updates while I was away. My father became delirious and disoriented. He fought with his nurses. He insisted on going home. But the hematoma fortunately remained stable, and my father was able to be discharged from the hospital before I returned from London.

His gait deteriorated over the next several days, however. By the time Harwinder and I took him to his neurosurgery follow-up appointment the following week, he could barely walk, his soles scraping against the warm asphalt as he shuffled unsteadily across the clinic parking lot that morning. I struggled to get him up the steps to the double doors, where an attendant was waiting with a wheelchair to whisk him away for a CT scan that had been scheduled for that morning.

This scan showed that the hematoma had substantially increased. There was now an almost one-centimeter rightward shift of my father's brain inside his skull. Because his brain had atrophied so much, the skull could still accommodate a few millimeters more of shift. But space was running out.* Once the brain was pushed up against the

* The excess space inside a skull holding an atrophied brain produces a suction effect that causes blood and fluid to fill up under the bone and within the ventricles, the brain's fluid-filled chambers. Matthew Baillie, an eminent Scottish pathologist, may have been the first to comment on this distinctive characteristic of the brains of individuals with dementia. "Under such circumstances, the ventricles are sometimes found enlarged in size and full of water," he wrote in his textbook *The Morbid Anatomy of Some of the Most Important Parts of the Human Body* in 1793, though he did not recognize that this enlargement was a sign of atrophy or dementia.

inner part of the skull, grievous and possibly irreversible injury could occur.

From the scan I took my father by wheelchair to the eighth floor of the neurological wing, where we met Dr. Jamie Ullman, the neurosurgeon who'd taken care of my father in the hospital when he was an inpatient the week before. She told me that the new gait difficulty and some of the other odd behaviors he'd displayed over the previous week (including pooping in the shower) were probably consequences of the expanding hematoma. Pressure on the frontal lobes from pooling blood could cause patients to lose their inhibitions, she said. Desires formerly kept under wraps could emerge, along with a debilitating lack of awareness of the inappropriateness of the behavior. "It can be very stressful," she said sympathetically, glancing at Harwinder.

After reviewing the CT scan, she said we had three options: drilling a hole in the skull to drain the hematoma; using a steroid, such as Decadron, to suppress tissue inflammation; or observing my father for another week to see if the hematoma began to resolve on its own. However, because of my father's rapidly worsening condition, she recommended surgery—a "decompressive craniectomy" that would remove a two-inch piece of skull to create a "window" for the hematoma to drain. The operation was potentially lifesaving, but it carried risks: damage to blood vessels, leakage of cerebrospinal fluid, infection, and even stroke. There could also be complications from general anesthesia, including ICU delirium. "He may need to be tied down" after the operation, Ullman said. "That itself carries risks."

I asked her what she would do if it were her father. As a physician, I had been asked this question many times. It seemed to distill everything that patients or their loved ones wanted to know in a crisis. And yet, even as I asked the question, I couldn't help but think that it conveyed distrust, skepticism, an implication that medical care was contextual, somehow different if you loved the patient more.

Ullman affirmed that she would choose surgery. So, after discussing it with my siblings, I agreed to proceed. The risks of the operation were dwarfed by the fact that my father could barely walk. If the hematoma got worse, he would undoubtedly become bedbound. We knew he wouldn't want to live his life that way. Our path, though fraught, was clear.

From the neurosurgery suite I took my father to the hospital admitting office, where they put a barcode on his wrist and used a laser to identify him like a grocery product. I signed a pile of forms on his behalf, mostly to satisfy privacy and other regulations. Then he was transferred to a third-floor step-down unit for observation until the surgery, planned for the following morning.

That evening, sitting at his bedside as nurses weaved in and out of the four-bed unit, I tried to force-feed him mashed potatoes and chicken strips, the last meal he could have before his operation, but he wouldn't eat. I gave him a few pieces of an orange, which he chewed for the sweetness but spit out. He nibbled disinterestedly on a candy bar, smearing the chocolate all over his white sheets. It had been almost two days since he'd properly eaten. His appetite had all but disappeared.

When I left at one in the morning, he was sleeping. His face, though drawn, still had hardly a wrinkle. He continued to appear two decades younger than his seventy-nine years. Apart from his brain, I realized, there really wasn't much that was physically wrong with him.

The operation took place at 7:30 the following morning, a Saturday. As planned, the chief of neurosurgery, a friend of my brother's, came in to do the case. It took about two hours. Dr. Narayan peeled back the skin and tissue overlying the back of my father's skull to reveal the bone. Next he used a drill and a saw to cut out a Post-it–sized piece of bone to drain the coagulated blood and allow my father's compressed brain to reexpand. Then the bone was replaced, and the wound was bandaged.

After a short stay in the postanesthesia care unit, my father was taken to a small room in the neurosurgical ICU, where at around eleven that morning I found him lying on his side, looking miserable as a nursing assistant kept close watch so he wouldn't pull out the thin tube that was taped to his scalp, draining bloody fluid.

He spent that night in fitful sleep. The following morning I found him struggling to sit on the bedside commode. "It's a shame," he cried.

"What's a shame?" I asked.

"This hospital," he replied. "Nothing works!"

He could have been talking about himself. His main problem after the operation wasn't the bleeding around his brain or the complications of the surgery as much as it was the breakdown of his elemental bodily processes, such as emptying of the bladder. Urinary retention was initially caused by the drugs used to deliver anesthesia, but it persisted for a variety of reasons, including pain medications, sedatives, and physical immobility. At times his bladder swelled to a dangerous size. Even so, he bitterly fought off nurses who attempted to catheterize him. "Please ma'am, don't do that," he'd start off politely. "Please, ma'am . . . it's painful!"

"We have to empty your bladder, Doctor."

"No!"

As Ullman had predicted, my father was soon wearing a Posey vest tied to the bed frame, shouting at the nurses to let him go free.

"You can't leave," I'd try to explain as he strained futilely against the cloth restraints.

"Why not?!"

"Because you fell, Dad. You had brain surgery."

Perplexed, he'd sit back, allowing for a temporary respite—until the tape in his brain rewound.

However, about a week into his postsurgical hospital stay, a head CT showed some improvement. The deviation across the midline of his skull had decreased from twelve millimeters to six. His brain was finally returning to a more normal shape.

The day before he was to be discharged, Harwinder, who had been staying with him for much of the day, took me aside in the ICU corridor.

"You brothers should come more often," she said. "I will be with him"—she'd agreed to stay with my father 24-7 until he recovered—"but a son is special. He wants to feel, My sons took time to visit me."

"You are right," I said, feeling chastened. "We have not been doing enough. On a scale from 1 to 100, we are probably a 25. Some sons keep their parents in their own home."

"On that count, you are a zero," she said coldly.

It took a moment to absorb the blow.

"Just come more often," she continued sympathetically, appearing sorry for her remark. "When you don't come for a few days, he says, 'Look at my kids, they don't come to see me. When a person gets old, no one cares anymore.' He raised you, he made you a doctor. If you don't do your duty, we will all feel it."

The following day, my father went home. The hospital team had recommended a stint at a rehabilitation facility, but it was obvious that my father was not going to do well in another institutional setting, so we declined.

That night, we met for dinner at his house. My father was in my mother's old recliner in the living room quietly watching TV, while the rest of the family, including my sister, who'd flown in from Minneapolis, was seated at the dining table. Midway through dinner, he finally spoke. "Where is your mom?" he said. He hadn't mentioned her in months.

My brother quickly got up. "Mom isn't here," Rajiv said.

"Where is she?" my father demanded.

I put down my utensils and went over to him. "Dad," I said quietly, kneeling beside him. "Mom died three years ago."

He looked at me like I was crazy. "She flew with me to this place one month ago," he cried. "Call the airline. Ask them, 'There was a passenger. What happened to her?'"

I started to speak, but Rajiv interrupted me. "We'll call the airline tomorrow," he said. "Right now, the plane is still in flight."

I shot him a hard look, but my father seemed just fine with this plan. "Okay, please remember," he said to Rajiv.

After the meal, which my father mostly refused to eat, Harwinder and I took him upstairs. First, we took him to the bathroom, where he quickly brushed his teeth. Then we got him into bed. "Keep moving," I said as he backed unsteadily toward the mattress. "More, more. Okay, sit down. Good. Now turn and lie down."

I drew the comforter over him and pulled up the steel side rails that we'd had installed while he was in the hospital. I tried to get him to raise his head to allow me to shove another pillow under it to make him more comfortable, but he couldn't be bothered. Keep your chin stiff and weather the blows: it was what he'd been doing his whole life.

I switched on the television and lowered the volume so he could sleep. He was staring up at the ceiling, his eyes blinking rapidly. The staples around the scar on his skull occasionally glinted in the moonlight. "Sandeep," he said hesitantly. "When I go home . . . can you give me the number for your mom?"

"We'll talk about it later, Dad. Now just try to get some rest."

"Can you just give me her number?"

"He has said this before," Harwinder whispered.

"And what did you tell him?"

"What could I tell him?" she replied, throwing her hands up. "I told him the truth."

"Please, Sandeep," my father said, reaching out to touch my arm. "I just want to talk to her."

"Dad, that number is gone," I said, flinching. "I told you before, Mom died three years ago. Nothing we do or say is going to bring her back."

"How do you know?"

"We went to her funeral."

"You went to her funeral?!" He tried to sit up, but he could barely raise his head off the pillow.

"So did you."

"I did not," he roared. "You are such a man! You are sitting here and you don't even know where your mom is."

When I went back downstairs, Rajiv and Suneeta were sitting in the living room discussing my father's care plan. "What more is there to talk about?" Rajiv said as I went to the kitchen to get a glass of water. "Harwinder is going to work on Sundays."

"We need to tell her to spend quality time with him," my sister urged. "He is at a critical time. He needs to use his brain, or he is going to get worse."

"You have unreasonable expectations," Rajiv said dismissively. "We are not going to make him better now."

My sister glared at him. "If we don't engage his brain, he will get worse," she said with forced coolness. It was the usual calm before the storm.

"I am sorry to say, but you are clueless," Rajiv replied. "Dad's condition has changed. I have no idea what care he will need, but I guarantee you that Harwinder alone won't be enough. So please don't criticize her, and let's keep things going for as long as possible."

"Criticize her?" Suneeta said, raising her voice. "I have been the one begging her to stay or we will have to send him to a nursing home. Trust me, she is only staying because of me, not you! In fact, she thinks you both fucking suck! She says she's never seen sons like you, and she has never seen sisters-in-law like mine. So think before you say something!"

"We are not going to send Dad to a nursing home regardless," I said, sitting down. "We will spend the money for home care."

"The reason I'm saying nursing home is because she told me today that she is only going to stay for a few more months," Suneeta said. "So obviously we will have to consider a nursing home if she leaves. He can't use a phone. He is peeing all over the house. He can't put his—"

"She is not the only caregiver," I said, interrupting her. "We can find an agency that specializes in dementia. We will have to pay, but we would have to pay for a nursing home, too."

She shook her head in frustration, her eyes welling. "I can't believe this is happening," she said. "I am so far away, and I can't do anything."

"This is why I never cried after Mom died," Rajiv said.

"Why didn't you?!" she spat out, her eyes afire.

"I was sort of relieved," Rajiv replied evenly. "I saw the writing on the wall. I loved Mom as much as you guys, but she was suffering, and my biggest fear was that she would break a hip and be in pain."

"That doesn't mean that you don't cry when she dies," my sister said savagely.

"I am not wearing it as a badge of honor; I am just telling you the truth." He put his arm around her, his tone now softer. "What are your expectations, Sun?" he said. "They need to be realistic. Peace, painlessness, and dignity."

"I know," she sobbed.

When I went back upstairs, Harwinder was still sitting with my father. His eyes were now closed, his head tipped back, nostrils flaring as he lightly snored. Harwinder had arranged two pillows on either side of his head to keep him from irritating his wound. One had slipped down and was partially covering his mouth. I put my hand on it. A few more pounds of pressure, I allowed myself to think, and this long saga would be over.

I removed my hand. My father opened his eyes. "Oh, you've come," he said.

"Yes, I came, Dad. Do you need anything?"

He shook his head. "Did you bring Pia?"

I couldn't help but smile. "Yes, she is downstairs."

He took a deep breath and settled back onto the pillow. We sat in silence, his eyes now open. In the ambient light I could see his lips moving. The sound coming from them was faint, indistinct.

"What are you saying, Dad?"

He shook his head but continued to murmur.

"He sings this song sometimes," Harwinder said. I asked her what the name of it was, but she didn't know.

"What are you singing, Dad?"

He didn't respond, but his lips continued to flutter slowly. "Chan . . . kitthan . . . guzari . . . ," Harwinder finally made out. "He is singing to the moon."

Later that night, I Googled the lyrics. They were from an old Punjabi love song.

"My dear, where did you spend the night?" the song's translation read.

> I was wide awake with your memories,
> And with the stars in the sky.
> You forgot about your promise, that
> You would come quickly.
> That is what you said before leaving.
> Oh moon, where are you?
> Oh moon, where did you spend the night?

IF YOU DON'T KNOW MATH,
THAT IS NOT MY PROBLEM

A few nights after returning home from the hospital, my father stayed awake yelling for me, my mother, my sister (who'd flown back to Minneapolis), and Harwinder, who spent a few hours in the middle of the night hiding in the guest bedroom, trying to avoid the old man shuffling in a rage around the house. On video I saw him wake her up at three o'clock in the morning. "We have to go," he cried. "We will miss the train!" He started to throw things on the bed. "That woman who works for me. Where is she?"

"I am that woman," Harwinder replied, but he did not believe her. When he asked where his wife was, she told him that his wife had died many years ago. That was when he threw Harwinder out of the house. But, as per her usual routine, she snuck back inside and hid in the guest room for a couple of hours until he got tired pacing back and forth in the upstairs hallway and eventually fell asleep.

By the following morning, a cloudy Saturday, he was better. A visiting nurse was scheduled to come over to assess his home care needs, so, just before nine o'clock, I drove up to the house.

He was still in bed when I arrived. I took him to the bathroom to wash up. He limped up to the toilet and urinated on the toilet seat.

Then he went to the sink to wash his hands. Peering out the window into a neighbor's yard, he said, "Some people keep a canal."

"That's a swimming pool, Dad," I said, unable to help myself.

"Yes, but they have a canal, too," he said vaguely. This time I stopped myself from correcting him.

He sat on the edge of the bathtub as we struggled to take off his boxers. I turned on the faucet in the shower. With some effort, I got him to sit on the chair we had placed in the stall. I covered his scalp with a clear plastic bag to prevent water from getting on the stapled wound. Then, after wetting the skin, I lathered up his naked body. To wash off the soap, I poured warm water from a plastic cup onto his back. "Is it okay?" I asked, just like when he used to bathe me after we went swimming at the Y.

"It's nice and warm," he said appreciatively.

After he was finished with his bath, I took him over to the sink to get a shave. He'd been complaining that his razor wasn't working, and now I understood why: the plastic protective cap was still on. With the cap removed and a few brisk strokes, white dollops studded with beard shavings fell into the sink. "I think it's working!" he said excitedly as the scraping turned into a smooth glide.

Before we left the bathroom, I made him gulp down his morning pills. "What day will we start with tomorrow?" I asked, showing him the pillbox.

"Sandeep, please don't police me," he said tiredly.

"Dad, what's the day today?"

"What's today? I don't know." He looked over at the calendar hanging on the wall. "What's the day today?"

"You tell me."

"Friday?"

I shook my head. "Monday?" he said.

"No, it's Saturday, because I don't have to work today. So which pills will you take tomorrow?"

He pointed to the left-most well.

"That's Monday. We're talking about *tomorrow* morning."

"I don't know," he said, giving up.

"What day comes after Saturday?"

"Sunday."

"So which pills are you going to take?"

"This one," he said finally, pointing to the proper well.

I told myself to be patient. It *was* confusing. The days in a week cycle in a circle, but a pillbox is linear. We take for granted that our brains can reconcile these disparate concepts, but it's easy for us only because our brains make it so. Be grateful, I reminded myself, that yours is still doing its job.

Back in the bedroom, now showered and shaved, my father appeared more relaxed.

"So, what is your program?" he said brightly.

"No program, Dad. I'll be here for a few hours."

"You mean here with me?" he said with an impish grin. "Gosh, I am lucky."

I laughed. "You're in a good mood," I said.

"Seeing you puts me in a good mood."

"Then I should come more often."

"Yes, that's right, young man," he belted out jovially.

Standing with a towel around his waist, he started to put on his boxers.

"No, sit down. Sit down to put on your . . . Stop!"

"What is it?" he demanded, taken aback.

"You're putting both feet in the same hole."

"Putting in the same one?"

"Yes, you can't do that." I made him sit on the bed and called out to Harwinder for help. When she appeared, she told me to step aside; she would dress him. She'd been doing it, she reminded me, for more than a year.

Once he was dressed, I helped him down the stairs. I stood behind him, my hands at the ready, as he leaned forward, both hands on the railings, and slowly made his way down the steps.

"Those steps are going to be a problem," Rajiv said from the living room. "This was never a good house for parents with brain disease."

The bell soon rang, and Rajiv went to open the front door. It was Barbara, a visiting nurse who'd been scheduled at hospital discharge to perform my father's home assessment. Carrying a leather bag, she stepped into the foyer. She looked over at the living room, immediately beginning to take the measure of the house. My brother showed her to a seat at the dining table.

We talked for about half an hour while my father sat quietly and listened. She told us that Medicare would pay for home care, including physical therapy, for which my father obviously qualified, but only in the short term until he got stronger. For long-term coverage, my father would have to apply for Medicaid. To meet the financial eligibility criteria, we would have to create a trust to legally shelter his assets. Even so, there was a waiting period, and at the end of it she could not guarantee that we would be able to keep Harwinder as the primary caregiver, at least not full-time. My siblings and I had already decided that we would take no decision that would compromise the relationship Harwinder had developed with our father. So Medicaid, I told Barbara, was not an option.

She asked about my father's condition prior to the tumble. I told her that until a month ago he'd been walking around the neighborhood by himself and even driving to Trader Joe's with Harwinder. She shot me a disbelieving look. "It goes without saying," she whispered, "that you should now take away his keys."

We had decided to do this even before the spill. Of all the children, I'd held out the longest, hoping to preserve his freedom even as we gradually whittled down the distance he was allowed to drive. The breaking point had come about a month before his fall, when, while navigating on a busy road, he'd asked Harwinder, who'd never learned how to drive, which was the gas pedal and which was the brake. Two weeks later, he hit a neighbor's car while backing out of the driveway. (He denied this.) That was when Rajiv put the old Audi up for sale.

I took Barbara upstairs to inspect my father's bedroom. She pointed out potential slip hazards, such as the bathroom rug, and provided a checklist for preventing trips and falls. We would have to install grab bars in the shower, she said, as well as supervise my father when he bathed. He was never to be left alone in the bathroom, at least not until he regained his strength and balance. When I informed her that neither he nor Harwinder would be comfortable with this plan, she said that she would apply for a male aide, if possible, to assist him with showering, but that there was a long waitlist; it was one of the home-care needs that was hardest to fill. "How often does he take a shower?" she asked.

"Just once," I answered.

"Once a week?" she said hopefully.

"Once a day," I said sharply.

Before she left, she said she would request as many home services as were available, including physical and occupational therapy, though budgets were tight and she couldn't make any promises. In any case, she said, someone would reach out to us on Monday. (My father ended up having a female shower aide for about a week, until he fired her, and home visits from a physical therapist for about two weeks.)

After Barbara and Rajiv walked out, I also got up to go. "You'll walk every day?" I said to my father from the front door.

"No," he replied.

"You'll walk every other day, then?"

"Yes."

"Okay, I'll come every other day to walk with you." It was a critical time, I reminded him. He would have to participate fully in his own physical rehabilitation if he wanted to get better. "Remember, life is a struggle," I said, and we both laughed as it occurred to us—or perhaps just to me—that I sounded just like him.

In the months that followed, my father did get stronger. He was soon able to go to the bathroom on his own, and he eventually went back to taking short walks in the neighborhood. Though he didn't remember the particulars of his fall—whether, in fact, he had even fallen—for weeks he was afraid to go outside. So he must have remembered something, even if he couldn't tell me what it was.

Despite the physical improvements, however, he continued to deteriorate mentally. By that summer he was having bizarre delusions that would stay with him in one form or another for the remainder of his life.

"Does Hicksville have a Pusa Institute?" Suneeta texted Rajiv and me one Sunday afternoon. "I think Dad must mean the library. I found one on Jerusalem Road, which is 1.7 miles from his house. Can one of you take him there?"

"The Pusa Institute is in New Delhi," Rajiv responded. "It's where he used to work."

It became the new routine, his waking up from his nap every afternoon insisting he needed to go to the Pusa Institute on Mathura Road. Then, in the middle of the night, he'd get up and insist on brushing his teeth or taking a shower because the Indians who'd come from India had settled in a colony nearby, and he wanted to go and visit them. Most evenings he'd tell me he wanted to go home.

"What do you mean, you want to go home, Dad? *This—*"

"Sandeep! When I say I want to go home, you should know which home I want to go to."

"But you live here."

"I don't!"

"Where do you live, then? These are Mom's pictures! This is your computer."

We didn't know whether the subdural hematoma had expanded, but we did not want to repeat the CT scan to find out. (What were we going to do if it had?) Maybe the head injury had accelerated his Alzheimer's, as I'd read could happen, or maybe the dementia had simply progressed on its own timeline. Whatever the reason, I knew my father's psychosis portended a grave prognosis. Study after study in the literature shows that the presence of hallucinations or delusions in patients with dementia increases the risk of disability, institutionalization, and death.

Additional peculiarities cropped up that summer, too. My father's sense of hot and cold went awry—maybe because the disease process was affecting his hypothalamus, the area of the brain that controls body temperature. He would wear a sweater and jacket when it was one hundred degrees outside. Harwinder hid his winter clothes in the basement so he wouldn't suffer heatstroke.

Other behavior was equally bizarre. He would get a ride from Harwinder's cousin to the bank to check his balance and transactions, most of which he hadn't made and none of which he recognized. He'd sometimes stay for hours, shouting at tellers, demanding explanations, while Harwinder and her cousin waited outside or went and did some nearby shopping. "This is the worst period," Rajiv said, "because he thinks he can comprehend, but he can't."

Dr. Gupta, the psychiatrist, suggested we get a second opinion from Dr. Angela Scicutella, a geriatric psychiatrist he respected, so Harwinder and I took my father to see her one blazing afternoon in late July 2019. We parked in a run-down section of Queens near homes with chain-link fences and rusted pickup trucks, walked into a ramshackle building, and took an elevator up to her office. Scicu-tella greeted us herself in the waiting room and took us to the back. She was a wiry, middle-aged woman with short brown hair and a pleasingly direct manner, at least compared to Gupta's. Displayed prominently on her desk was a plastic model of a human brain, which sat in front of us as my father took a seat between Harwinder and me on a small couch. He was polite as introductions were made, but I could tell he just wanted to go home.

Scicutella began the interview by asking about my father's recent history. I told her about his fall three months prior, his subsequent surgery, and his recent history of paranoia and delusions—including the belief that my mother, who'd died more than three years earlier, was still alive. "Oh gosh," she murmured sympathetically. My father stayed quiet, interrupting only once to ask whom we were talking about.

"We're talking about you, Dad."

"When he says, 'We are talking about you,' are you okay with that?" Scicutella asked. "How does that make you feel?"

"I don't know," my father said.

She asked him a few personal questions, but his answers were nonsensical. He said we moved to the United States during the par-tition of India in 1947. He claimed he had two daughters, not one. One of them was a girl named Suneeta who was fourteen or fifteen years old.

"And how old are you, Doctor?"

"Thirty-two."

"And what was your job?"

"I forgot," he said quickly.

"You did cytogenetics, Dad. You wrote books."

He started laughing. "He is trying to flatter me."

As he spoke, I noticed he was making repetitive movements with his jaw. For a while I'd thought that they were a side effect of one of his mood-stabilizing medications, but Scicutella now told me that people living with dementia often develop perseverative behaviors, such as rubbing of the skin or grinding of the teeth, which are likely a sign of frontal lobe dysfunction. The behaviors are difficult to stop, she said, in part because patients are usually unaware of them and have little insight into their damaging effects. You can put creams or gloves on their hands, for example, yet patients still develop deep lacerations and sometimes even require antibiotics for wound infections.

During cognitive testing, my father said it was 1939. The season, he said, was September. He was able to repeat the words "banana," "tiger," and "honesty" immediately after they were spoken but could not remember any of them after three minutes (though he got "banana" after some prompting). He correctly repeated the phrase "above, beyond, and below." When shown pictures, he was able to name a pencil, a watch, and a crown, but other pictures elicited only nonspecific responses such as "furniture," "animal," and "bird." His semantic knowledge had deteriorated. He answered that a nickel was worth ten cents.

Scicutella asked him to write a sentence, as Dr. Gordon had asked more than four years earlier, though now with different results.

"What sentence?" he said testily. He'd been there for almost an hour, and his patience was wearing thin.

"You decide," Scicutella replied.

"Ma'am, you are confusing me. Write a sentence about what?"

"I want you to decide. Whatever's on your mind."

He stared at the blank sheet for almost a minute. "I don't know what you want me to write," he said.

"Anything, Dad. Just write whatever comes to your—"

"Okay, leave it," he interrupted, setting the paper aside. So we moved on.

It was clear that his disease had progressed rapidly since the visit to Dr. Gordon the past winter. I'd been reading about blood tests being developed to detect Alzheimer's at an early stage, before significant brain damage has occurred. These tests would pick up signatures of beta-amyloid and tau protein in the serum before symptoms were evident. Eventually, experts were predicting, the tests might even be available for home use. Obviously, there would be risks associated with such testing—discrimination by employers and insurers, stigmatization by family and friends, and the costs and burdens of downstream verification—but the benefits of detecting dementia early were clear to me that July afternoon. If we had known about his condition earlier, my father could have retired sooner and enjoyed more time with my mother. He could have engaged in end-of-life planning conversations with us while he was still able. But the possibility that he would have any say in such talks had long been lost.

After the formal testing was completed, Scicutella picked up a sponge ball and tossed it to my father, who did not react. He didn't know what to do with the ball on the floor, so she instructed him to throw it back to her. He did. She caught it and threw it back. Then he caught it. Back and forth the ball went over the desk. Before long I noticed my father was smiling.

"We believe in intellectual and social stimulation, no matter what stage of the disease," Scicutella told me as they continued to play catch—which, despite all of his forgetting, my father clearly had not forgotten how to do. "I do this with all my patients. It's good for hand-eye coordination, and it gives them an activity."

To promote more activity in his life, she suggested, it might be worthwhile to enroll my father in a day program. There were a couple good ones locally—one at the Jewish Community Center in Greenvale and another at the Long Island Alzheimer's Foundation in Westbury, near his house. The program would give him an opportunity to play games, listen to music, and meet and interact with other patients. When I expressed skepticism over whether my father would go along with this plan, Scicutella said, "A lot of people say the same thing: 'My mother isn't a joiner,' 'My father isn't social.' Well, he's cooperating with me right now. Now, maybe it's because of the white coat, I get it, but I've had patients who push the ball away. He's at least trying." She was hopeful that a little more activity in his day might head off my father's episodes of confusion. Until then, she was going to prescribe Seroquel, an antipsychotic, morning, noon, and night.

"Are you okay with everything we're talking about?" she said, turning to my father.

He thought about it for a moment. "You are telling numerous questions and answers," he said, summing up his experience of the afternoon. "The only question I have is, Will it be of any use?" A trace of the old scientist, cutting to the core of the matter, was still there.

"I am looking to make your days a bit easier, Doctor," Scicutella responded. "I recommend some exercises at a program to get you out of the house."

"One has to go for several days?" he asked.

"No, just once or twice a week."

He shrugged. "To my mind, it is ridiculous, but you may feel differently. My only question is, Will it help?"

A few weeks later, on a sunny day after a drenching rain, I pulled up to the house to take my father to his first day session at the Long Island Alzheimer's Foundation in Westbury. He had been dressed smartly by Harwinder that morning in a gray pinstriped suit and a paisley tie. After much encouragement, he seemed to be looking forward to the experience. Harwinder, too, had high hopes, not the least of which were for the three hours of respite the program would afford her three times a week.

The Alzheimer's center was on a busy thoroughfare near cheap motels and an Olive Garden. In the lobby, I perused informational pamphlets on support groups and companion services while we waited for an escort to take us in. Before long, a bespectacled social worker named Melissa came out and led us to a meeting room, where she served us coffee—she smiled when my father tried to drink it by sucking on the plastic stirrer—and gave us a brief introduction to the facility. When she was finished, she gave a brochure each to my father, Harwinder, and me. "Long Island Alzheimer's Foundation," my father read aloud. He inserted the brochure into the sheaf of papers he'd brought with him.

Since I'd already informed Melissa about my father's condition over the phone, she took us down the hall to where the program was taking place. There were three rooms in use. In the first, participants with mild dementia were sitting at a large table doing crossword puzzles. An aide was circulating, checking on their progress and offering encouragement: "Clean as a—" "Still waters run—" On a table near the door were stacks of books and more word games. It looked like the bingo room at any nursing home. "We don't think this would be the best fit," Melissa said.

In an adjoining room, the elderly participants were sitting stooped in wheelchairs. The room was devoid of sound and movement, apart from that of an aide who'd been sitting quietly but now waved to say hello. The room reminded me of the memory ward where my grandmother had spent the last two years of her life. I was relieved to hear Melissa say that my father had been assigned to the third room.

When we entered, Juliette, a young counselor, welcomed us. She was dressed informally in a red sweat suit and sneakers, with a red bandanna tied to her head. Introducing herself, she said that she had been working at the center for a year but had been doing home health care and dementia companionship for almost six years. "We do many things here," she said brightly, showing my father to a seat at a long table. "Talk, play music, watch videos. We can do show-and-tell."

They were doing "art therapy" that morning: coloring in animal figures with crayons. Someone passed my father a drawing of a turkey along with a brown crayon and asked him to color it in, making sure to keep the marks within the outline. My father picked up the crayon but seemed unsure of what to do. He made a short streak with the crayon and set it down.

"This is good for you, Dad," I said, trying to encourage him.

"Come, on, Doctor," Juliette piped in. "You can give this to your grandson."

At my father's insistence, Harwinder sat down next to him, and he got to work. "We try to discourage the aides," Juliette whispered as we stepped into the hallway. "That way he doesn't have a crutch."

"It seems he isn't too excited for this activity," I said apologetically.

"He may be protecting himself because he doesn't know how to do it," she said. "Does he like sports? We could give him a Yankees logo instead."

"He was a scientist," I explained. "I'm not sure he understands the point of it."

When we went back inside, my father had put down the crayon. A teddy bear had been placed in front of him, and one of the aides was asking him if he wanted to hold it. "Sandeep, I think we should go," he said.

"Let's give it a chance, Dad," I admonished. "They have many activities."

Juliette asked him what else he might like to do.

"He's good at math," I offered. "Dad, what's twenty-seven plus eighteen?"

"What? Forty-five," he replied quickly.

"So, let's try something different," Juliette said, smiling and taking a seat. She took out an iPad and opened an arithmetic app. "Can you help me with some math?"

"What?" my father said.

"I'm not very good at math. Can you help me?"

"If you don't know math, that is not my problem. There are many teachers."

"But I want *you* to help me. Your son said you were very smart. Can you help me with this one? Negative four times negative three."

"Twelve."

The ring on the app said he got it right. "Good! Now, what's eighty-one divided by nine?"

They did a few more problems, most of which he answered correctly, but he was getting irritated. "Why are you asking me these questions?" he demanded.

"Because you're supposed to teach me math," Juliette responded.

"For free?!" he cried.

Having noticed that she'd been playing some R&B on her phone, I mentioned that my father enjoyed Marvin Gaye. At my request, she put on "Sexual Healing."

The transformation was almost immediate. My father had been sitting, arms folded, legs crossed, in a posture of irritation, but he was soon nodding agreeably to the music. Juliette asked him to dance. At first, he said no, but with some encouragement he stood up. He extended his hands stiffly and allowed her to grab them and sway him from side to side. *Baaay-by*, the song went. *I can't hold it much longer . . . It's getting stronger and stronger . . .* "See, you're learning some dance moves," she said. She held up her arms and did a twirl, brushing up against him. "That's good, young lady," my father murmured. "You are so good."

After the song was over, she tried to get him to do arts and crafts again, but he said he was tired. I thought it best to end the session on a high note, so after she finished drawing a butterfly for him, we left.

In my car, he was quiet. "So you didn't like the place?" I asked him.

"No," he replied.

I turned on the engine and backed out of the lot.

"What is the name of this place?" he asked me.

I passed him the brochure he'd tucked into his papers. "What does it say?" I asked him.

"Long Island . . . Foundation," he said, skipping the word "Alzheimer's."

"What was that?"

Shaking his head, he dropped the brochure on my lap. "Long Island Foundation," he said again.

I turned onto the main road to go home. "So, do you want to try it again next week?"

He put up his hand, indicating for me to stop talking.

"Come on, Dad. Don't give up so quickly. She was a nice girl. She danced with you."

"She was a duffer," he said acidly. "She did not know even simple math."

13

YOU'RE MY FAMILY

Alzheimer's disease is often divided into seven stages. My father was at stage 3 (mild decline) when he arrived on Long Island in the summer of 2014. At this stage, a person already has cognitive difficulties. He may be unable to perform at his job as he once did, or he may forget names or where he put personal possessions. Though formal testing can detect such impairment, day-to-day observation by family members often cannot distinguish it from usual age-related cognitive changes.

From this stage, my father's disease progressed steadily. He was at stage 4, moderate dementia, by the winter of 2015–2016, just before my mother died. By then, he had clear symptoms of Alzheimer's (or, more likely, mixed-type) dementia: disabling short-term memory loss; inability to manage his finances or pay his bills. He was beginning to forget important details of his personal history.

He reached stage 5 (moderate-to-severe dementia) in the months after my mother died. No doubt the loss of his life partner and the ensuing social isolation accelerated his decline. At stage 5, patients begin to need help with most daily activities. They have difficulty dressing appropriately. They often cannot walk alone outside their homes because they get lost. Paranoia and disorientation can also set in. My father felt suspicious of his children's motives, particularly regarding his finances. He also had a paralyzing loss of insight into his difficulties and need for daily help. However, he was still able to perform the basic activities of daily living, such as bathing and toileting independently. Most importantly, he still recognized his family.

Stage 6 came on rapidly after his fall and hospitalization. At this stage he required constant supervision. He sometimes seemed unaware of where he was. He didn't recognize people other than his closest friends or relatives in photographs. He went to sleep as soon as it got dark, perhaps because the brain centers that control the sleep-wake cycle were damaged. He began to experience loss of bladder control, too, frequently wetting himself at night, requiring a diaper.

By the fall of 2020, amid the Covid pandemic, he'd started wandering. It was a consequence of his brain degeneration—most people living with dementia do eventually wander—but I couldn't help but think that his constant desire to be someplace else also reflected nostalgia for an earlier time when he was independent. He had never been happy living on Long Island near his sons. The plans he'd conceived for himself and my mother in their old age had fallen apart. Though careful, anticipatory, and farsighted, even he had not foreseen the course of his physical and mental decline or just how much his children would change and outgrow the promises we'd made.

At stage 7, the final stage of Alzheimer's, patients need assistance with virtually every aspect of daily living. They lose the ability to respond to their environment. They often lose the ability to swallow or manage their own oral secretions. They have difficulty standing up, so they develop bedsores and urinary tract infections; or they fall and break their bones and become bedridden and contract pneumonia. I would often remember what Dr. Day at Washington University in St. Louis had told me. "In the final stages, all dementias look alike," he'd said. "The whole brain is affected. Patients generally can't speak."

The final sequence of end-stage disabilities seems to reverse the order of a young child's first developmental milestones, as one would expect with the progressive erasure of the most fundamental networks in the brain. As David Shenk wrote in his masterful book *The Forgetting*, "Alzheimer's unravels the brain almost exactly in the reverse order as it develops from birth." Initially, patients can no longer walk unaided. Then they can no longer sit up without assistance. Next, they lose the ability to smile. And finally they cannot hold up their own heads.

None of his children wanted to see their father progress to this final stage of the disease. But what were we willing to do to prevent such an end?

It was October 2020, and he was getting ready to go to the "station" to take the train to Kanpur to meet his mother and his older brother, Suraj. Suitcases were out, clothes littered on the bed. After a few days of respite from the madness, the house was a mess again.

"There is no train, Dad," I said again.

"There *is* a train," he shouted.

Wearing boxers and a white T-shirt, he was peering out the living-room window as though performing some sort of reconnaissance. At that moment he looked completely mad.

"Where are my pants?" he called out to Harwinder.

"Tell him they went for dry cleaning," she said from the kitchen.

"They are being dry-cleaned," I said.

"You gave them for dry cleaning?" he asked me suspiciously.

"Yes," I said. "The store is closed. It's Sunday." (It was Tuesday.)

He turned to Harwinder. "I have no other pants?"

"No," she replied. (At least none outside the boxes of clothes she'd hidden in the basement to keep him from leaving).

He turned away in disgust. "I will go like this then."

I got up from the sofa, afraid that I'd have to physically restrain him. "Dad, I am really worried about you. I can't let you go out like this."

"Sandeep, you worry and keep sitting here! Keep worrying and worrying—"

"It's raining, Dad. Do you even know where you're going?"

"I need another shirt, Harwinder. Come on, let's go!"

"I am not going," she said. "I told you ten times, I have to cook dinner. You go wherever you want, but I am staying here."

He turned to me, his tone softer. "Sandeep, will you come with me, please?"

"If you tell me where you're going, Dad. I don't know where you're going."

"I told you, the station."

"What do you want to do at the station? The station is where the trains—"

"Okay, don't come," he shouted, before I could finish. "You are such a man! 'What do you want to do at the station?'" he repeated mockingly. "Call a taxi, Bubby," he commanded. "Tell them to come now."

Harwinder held up her phone. "I just called. They said we don't send drivers at night. They will start again in the morning time." She glanced at me. "Maybe you can take him around a little in your car," she said quietly.

"What are you saying?" he shouted.

"Nothing, Uncle, we're just talking," she said tiredly, before going back to the kitchen to start preparing dinner.

In his compulsion to wander, my father was no exception. Two out of three people with dementia will eventually roam. Nearly half of those who are not found within twenty-four hours face serious injury or death.

In 2007, in Obu City, Japan, a ninety-one-year-old man with severe dementia who was under the care of his ailing wife was killed by a moving train after wandering away from his home. Citing the cancellation or delay of multiple trains, the Central Japan Railway Company actually sued the family of the man for damages, obtaining a judgment of ¥7.2 million (about $65,000) for compensation. Though the ruling was eventually dismissed by the Japanese Supreme Court, the case started a national conversation on dementia care in Japan, which has one of the world's largest populations of older adults as well as the highest proportion of those living with dementia.

In 2014, the Japanese government launched its "Orange Plan," a set of measures to provide sustainable long-term care for dementia patients. One initiative was the community-based SOS Wanderer Network to monitor the movement of dementia patients and reduce the risks associated with wandering. Other strategies included GPS and radio-frequency tracking devices, as well as a waterproof bar-code sticker affixed to a person's fingernail that police could use to access personal information, such as a home address. Such technologies raise all sorts of ethical questions about how to respect privacy and dignity while ensuring safety, questions that are complicated by demented individuals' diminished ability to consent to surveillance. In America, however, these issues are not at the forefront of dementia discourse because the responsibility for wandering patients continues to be borne almost entirely by their families.

By the time my brother showed up after work, my father was sitting at the dining table, a bit calmer but still insisting that he needed to make his train.

"The train to where, Dad?" Rajiv said. "Kanpur? Do you know where Kanpur even is?"

"Again, you are going back to the same questions, testing me," my father said bitterly.

"Who is in Kanpur?" Rajiv said, raising his voice. "There is no one left. Everyone is dead! Suraj, Kali, Sumitra, Mom, they're all dead. We are the only ones left. You, me, Sandeep, and Suneeta."

"You're messing up your house," I said, piling on. "You took the pictures off the wall." There were numerous holes where he had pried out the hanging studs. "Look!" I unlatched the suitcase on the floor. A jumble of garments exploded out of it. "You messed up your clothes. They were put away nicely."

"Harwinder did it."

"You forced her to do it."

"I did not."

"You did, Uncle," she said from her perch on the stairs. "You tried to hit me."

Looking back, I often wonder why I kept arguing with my father. In large part, I think, it was out of respect. I wanted to believe that he could act with reason—and therefore could respond to reason—even when his actions were seemingly irrational and meaningless. A part of it, no doubt, was denial. Though as a medical professional I understood clearly what was happening, as a son I continued to hold out hope for some insight or recovery. Of course, I was trapped in a certain cognitive bias, too. Like most loved ones of the mentally ill, I had no clue how else to communicate except through rational argument.

I picked up a yellow pad on the table. "Dad, where do you live?" I said with authority.

"Where do I live?" he replied quietly. "Fargo."

"You live in Fargo? What is this place?"

"This is part of Fargo."

"No, this is New York. Hicksville. Is this your house or not your house?"

"I don't know."

"It's your house. People live in their own house, right? Where do I live?"

"In your house."

"Right. In my own house. Where does Harwinder live? In your house," I continued quickly, before the thread of my argument was lost on him. "Because she doesn't have her own house. She lives here with you. Now, you were asking me, 'What is my destination?' It's right here. If you have business somewhere, you can go there, but you have no business in Kanpur. You have no business in Fargo. You have no place to stay."

I scribbled some instructions on a piece of paper and passed it to him.

"So, from here if I have to—"

"Read number one."

He glanced at the paper. "'You cannot go to Kanpur. You cannot go to Fargo. This is your house,'" he read.

"This is your house," I quickly continued. "If you want me to take you to Atlantic City for a little vacation, I can do that." He shook his head. "Do you want to visit Suneeta in Minneapolis?" I knew he didn't, which he confirmed with another shake of the head. "So, what is your destination? Your destination is here."

"So if I go to Kanpur, I'm coming back here?"

"If you go anywhere, you will always come back here, because this is your home. But there's nothing in Kanpur, Dad. It's dirty, it's hot, there are no proper toilet facilities. You left Kanpur to come to America. Now you want to go in the opposite direction?"

He nodded. He seemed to be finally understanding. He read the paper again. "'You cannot go to Kanpur. You cannot go to Fargo.'"

"Because you have no purpose there."

"But if I have to go there, how will I go?"

"If you must go, you will take a plane. But you don't have to go. You think you can take a plane by yourself?" He shook his head. "So you can't go there. Stop trying to pack. This is your house. Let's put this up on the wall so you don't forget."

He read it again. "'You cannot go to Kanpur. You cannot go to Fargo.'"

"Because you have no purpose there. Any other questions?"

"No, this is clear."

"So, are you going to keep packing?"

"Yes."

"Why?"

"Pack for Kanpur."

"What does it say here?"

"'You cannot go to Kanpur.' Yes, you are right. I got it."

"Anything else?"

"When I go from here, can I take a little snack with me?"

"To go where?"

He hesitated. "Anywhere."

"Yes, if you want to come to my house or go for a walk. But there is nowhere else for you to go. Do you understand?"

He turned to Harwinder. "From here, what are we going to take with us?"

"Nothing," she cried. "This is our house! We are going to stay here. He's been explaining to you for two hours."

"You've developed some dementia, Dad," Rajiv said. "This is a part of it. It is telling you to go somewhere."

"And you can't go anywhere," I said. "Because I will miss you."

That was when his breathing got heavy. "You will miss me?" He could barely get the words out. Then he broke down.

"Of course, I will miss you. I'm your son."

He quickly collected himself. Then he said, "Sandeep, when I go from here, how will—?"

"What is the number one thing on that paper?"

"'You cannot go to Kanpur.'"

"Keep reading."

"'You cannot go to Fargo.'"

"And what else?"

"'This is your house.'" He moved on to the next line. "'You will stay here forever.'"

By the time the winter of 2020–2021 arrived, my father was virtually bedbound, spending almost sixteen hours a day up in his room. He would be put to sleep before eight o'clock in the evening and not get up before nine the following morning. Rajiv and I began to spend more time at the house. Getting him downstairs for meals was a chore. He would spend maybe an hour or two downstairs after waking up, another hour or so after his afternoon nap, and then maybe another hour at dinnertime if he was in the mood. His appetite had waned, too. If he ate breakfast, he'd skip lunch; if he had lunch, sometimes he'd skip dinner. Instead of a full roti, he would eat half. He preferred sweetened liquids like Ensure and fruit juice.

Whatever dignity he retained was quickly vanishing. Because it would take some time to get him out of bed, he'd often urinate in his pajamas before making it to the bathroom. We finally put a diaper on him, which Harwinder would assiduously get up in the middle of the night to change to prevent infection. In the morning, she'd bathe him, lathering his skin, cleaning his crotch. She'd shave him, too, clipping his mustache, trimming his nails. If he didn't want to be bothered, he'd call her a bitch.

To keep him limber, she had him walk almost daily on the tread-mill. However, by winter he couldn't even make it onto the machine. He'd try to get on where the bar was; he couldn't make the calculation to move to the back where the path was open. If Harwinder tried to help him, he'd push her away. So that winter the treadmill went into hibernation, too.

Because he couldn't walk without assistance, the wandering—even the desire to wander—subsided. So did the rages. He started backing down whenever I spoke to him with authority. By the time the snows came and we were forced to hunker indoors, he had become almost placid. At support group meetings at the Alzheimer's Foundation, I learned that this passivity is common in the latter stages of dementia. "For a few years, my mother fought us on everything," a large, solid woman in her mid-fifties recalled at one gathering. "Now she doesn't know to fight anymore." By then I could have explained that the amygdala, the emotion-processing center in my father's brain, was degenerating. But knowing this took away none of the bittersweetness of watching my father's outbursts—perhaps even his emotion itself—disappear.

Before night arrived, Rajiv, Harwinder, and I would be exhausted. My father would insist that Harwinder sleep near him, so she took to sleeping on a mattress on the floor by his bed.

"Raj, are you sleeping?" he'd ask her.

"Yes," she'd reply.

"Can I get you some water?"

"No, I'm okay."

"Did you make my lunch? I have to go to the office early."

"I'll do it in the morning." In the morning, he would again call her Harwinder. But in the middle of the night, she became my dead mother.

One evening before Christmas, Rajiv asked me to go over to the house to plunge my father's toilet. He'd been doing it for the past several weeks, he told me, and he needed a break.

When I got to the house, I put on a mask, as I'd been doing for the past nine months, and Harwinder took me upstairs.

"What happened?"

"He messed up the toilet again, that's what happened," she said, obviously irritated. "I've been plunging it for half an hour. It got all over my shoes."

In the bathroom, dirty toilet water had collected into small puddles on the tile floor. I picked up the wooden plunger and dunked it into the bowl, brown water bubbling and frothing as I pumped. After about a minute I told Harwinder to pull the handle while I continued to plunge. Small pieces of turd immediately rose and streamed out onto the floor. I dropped the plunger when I started to retch.

"Just leave it and call a plumber," Harwinder said, laughing at the situation.

"There's something down there," I said. "Maybe he threw in the goddamn roll."

"Leave it," Harwinder said. "Big Sir"—her name for Rajiv—"said he would do it when he comes over."

"How is he going to do it if I can't do it?" I said, picking up the plunger again and starting to pump more aggressively. The plunger made loud vomiting noises. Dirty water droplets were flying everywhere. But just as I was about to give up, the water dropped suddenly, consumed in a sickening gurgle at the bottom of the bowl. Another flush and the toilet water was clear. I retched again. Harwinder giggled. "Congratulations," she said. "You saved yourself a hundred dollars."

After washing up, I went downstairs to find a dark yellow puddle lying by the front door. My father had urinated on the floor again while we were fixing the toilet. I quickly wiped up the mess with some paper towels.

Then I switched on CNN while Harwinder took my father upstairs for his predinner nap. On the television, Anderson Cooper was announcing the latest on Covid vaccines and the most recent public-health missteps by the Trump administration. I put my feet up on the coffee table and settled in to watch the news.

When Harwinder came back downstairs, she went to the kitchen to begin preparing dinner. In the window above the sink, a nearly full moon illuminated the snowy lawn. She started chopping vegetables. Lentils went into the pressure cooker. "Suneeta keeps telling me not to let him sleep so much," she said, her back to me. "When she comes, her eyes will be opened to the real situation."

"And what is that?" I asked, though I already knew what she was going to say.

She put down the knife and turned to me, drying her hands. "He is near the end. How long, no one can say. Whether it is two months, or six months, or six weeks, that only God knows. Whatever is written for him, that is how long he is going to live. Whatever sacrifices I have to make, that is what I am going to do."

She turned back to the chopping board.

"Why do you do it?" I asked her.

She started to cry. "I have no one now," she said, without looking at me. In the five years she'd been with us, her husband in India had passed away. With no green card, she hadn't been able to attend his funeral. Her children were grown, living in Canada. In the time since my mother's death, we had become her family. The experience of caregiving—the love and hate, courage and pity and frustration, the long periods of drudgery punctuated by craziness and emergencies and sometimes loving connection—we'd been through it all. But our time together was coming to an end.

"I think of him like a father," she said as the pressure cooker let off a plume of steam. "He gets angry, tries to hit me, says so many horrible words you want to cover your ears, but he loves me, too. He wants to know that I am close by. Sometimes he says, 'When I go, Bubby, will you come with me?'"

She wiped away her tears with the back of her hand. I asked her what she was going to do after he died. She said she would probably go to Canada to stay with one of her daughters.

"Will we ever meet?" I said, suddenly feeling a blanket of sadness settle over me.

"Of course," she reassured me. "We will call, FaceTime. When there is love, it will continue."

At seven thirty I went upstairs to bring my father down for dinner. He was lying on his side in the hospital bed he'd gotten a few months earlier, his face abutting the steel railing. With his red cap on and mustache trimmed, he still looked so much younger than his date of birth indicated. "You want to come downstairs for dinner, Dad?" I said encouragingly, but he said he wasn't hungry. He wanted to rest some more.

"Okay, I'll go then," I said. My work was done.

But he stopped me. "Can you stay for a little while?" he said.

I checked my watch. My family was surely waiting for me for dinner. "Anything you want to talk about, Dad?"

For a few moments, the room was still except for the low hum of a snowblower outside. Then he said quietly, "Can you take me with you?"

In his six and a half years on Long Island, he had never asked me to take him to my house. "What for, Dad?"

After a pause, he replied, "I want to apologize."

"Apologize for what?"

"For . . . the mistakes I have made."

"What mistakes, Dad?" Was he referring to the toilet?

"Many mistakes . . ."

"Today or throughout your life?"

"Today . . . and throughout my life."

"No, Dad, everything is fine," I tried to assure him. "You don't need to apologize to me. I am not angry with you."

"Please, Sandeep . . . I want to apologize to you . . . and others."

I've thought about this moment many times since his death. I'm still not sure what he meant to say or what he wanted to apologize for. Yet it was a moment I had been waiting for my whole life. A quiet bedroom. A snow-shrouded street. It was the way I'd always pictured it.

"Okay, apologize then."

"Apologize?"

"Yes."

"Okay. I am very, very . . . apologetic."

"I accept," I said immediately.

His face relaxed. "Thank you, sir. Thanks, my Bubboo."

"You're welcome." I made to go.

"Sandeep, can you lie with me?"

I gave a disbelieving laugh. "Come on, Dad, there isn't enough room for me!"

"There is room." He turned and struggled to move to the middle of the bed. "Come . . . we will make it work."

I went around to the far side of the bed where the disabled tread-mill still stood, pulled down the railing, and got into the bed with him. I switched on the flat-screen TV and muted the sound. On the bedside table were a lamp, some pill bottles, a roll of paper towels, and a few scientific reprints that I'd nonsensically placed there for his perusal. I absent-mindedly picked one of them up. "So, what else do you want to talk about?" I said.

"I love you, Sanja," he whispered. In all my years, I don't remember him ever telling me that.

"I love you, too."

"Can I ask you something?"

"Yes."

"Will you come and stay with me for some time?"

"Of course," I said automatically. "I have to go now, but I'll come again."

"If you can do it, I'll be very, very . . ."—he struggled to find the word—"apologetic. You're my family."

"Yes."

"And I love it."

I looked out the window. Evergreens weighed down by white powder cut through the gray sky. I had a terrible feeling that this would be his last winter.

"Anything else you want to talk about?" I said.

"Not really," he replied. "When I meet you again . . . I'll talk and talk and talk."

"Let's talk now," I said. "Who knows when we will meet again."

I switched on the lamp and passed him one of his reprints. "Oh, look at this," he said with vague interest.

"What is it?"

He laughed and slowly read the title: "Mapping population . . . for wheat stem . . . rust resistance."

"Did you do this work?"

"Not really."

"You used to work on wheat, right?" I pointed to a figure in the paper. "What is this?"

"This is . . . uh . . ."

"What are these black things?"

"These things? I don't know."

"They're chromosomes. Come on, you spent your life studying this stuff."

"Oh yes, chromosomes."

"What is this? Do you know?"

He hesitated. "It must be a wheat flower."

"Yes. These are all wheat plants. You used to grow them in the greenhouse."

"Yes."

"Do you miss those days?"

He shrugged. "Yes."

"Yes?"

"Yes."

"You liked work?"

"I liked . . . all these flowers and . . . you know . . ."

"You liked doing research."

"Yes. I liked to do research."

"Do you miss it?"

He nodded. "I miss it very much."

For the first time in months, it occurred to me that he wasn't unhappy. Because his decline had become so difficult to witness, I had hoped in my darkest moments that fall that he would die. But perhaps I was suffering over his condition more than he was. His world had shrunk, but so too had his desires, his perspective, his expectations of what constituted a worthwhile existence. Who was I to say how he should feel about his limited life? As long as he knew me and the people who loved him, perhaps that was all that mattered.

"Oh, you've come, Bubby," he said when Harwinder came in. "This is Sandeep. Have you met him?"

She looked at me and smiled. Dinner was ready, she said. She asked if he wanted to take it in bed or come downstairs.

"I will come with you," he said.

"You want to come downstairs?" I said skeptically.

"Yes," he replied. He tried to get up.

I brought him his walker, and we helped him out of bed. Holding tight to the roller, he was soon inching along the carpet that Rajiv had recently had installed. It took him a few minutes to get to the stairs, where he stopped. He was tired.

"I haven't told you something," he said, turning to Harwinder. "About Sandeep."

She smiled. "Tell me."

"He was the brightest student."

"Come on, Dad," I said impatiently. "Let's go."

We helped him down a step before he stopped again.

"Did I tell you: he's my most favorite."

"Hai hai," Harwinder cried, laughing.

I shook my head, bemused. We helped him down another step.

"I am very happy you came," he said to me, suddenly formal. "Once in a while . . . come to my house so we can eat together. Come with pleasure . . . and spend the night."

In the six and a half years since he'd moved to Long Island, I hadn't spent a single night at his house, I realized. "Okay," I said.

"You promise?"

"Yes, I will spend the night."

"The whole night?"

"Yes."

He laughed joyfully.

"Why are you laughing, Uncle?" Harwinder asked.

"He said he will spend the whole night here."

"Why not? He is your son."

"No," he cried. "He is not my son!"

"What am I then?"

Looking at me uncertainly, he said, "I think he is my nephew."

14

DON'T WORRY, THINGS WILL WORK OUT

There is no antidote against the opium of time, which
temporally considers all things: our fathers find their
graves in our short memories and sadly tell us how
we may be buried in our survivors.

—SIR THOMAS BROWNE, *Urn Burial*, 1658

It was a chilly Sunday afternoon in late February when my father
told me on the phone that he wanted to go out and have a dosa. "It's
raining," I said. "Are you sure?" He was. After two months of being
cooped up because of the cold weather and his increasing frailty, he
needed to get out of the house.

We struggled to make it across the parking lot at House of Dosas,
Harwinder and I holding my father on either side as the wind and
rain whipped our faces with a biting spray. Inside the restaurant, the
proprietor was pleasantly surprised to see us. He showed us, wearing
masks, to our usual table, where we ordered our usual meals. My father, in a festive green sweater, didn't eat much, but he seemed happy
to be sitting there watching the other patrons. By the time we made it

back to my car, it was getting dark. Raindrops pitter-pattered on the windshield as we drove home.

The following Wednesday, my father could not get out of bed. When I went over to see him that morning, he was moaning. Clenching his mouth shut, he wouldn't allow me to check his temperature orally. I tried giving him Advil and ciprofloxacin, an antibiotic he'd previously taken for a urinary tract infection—which I presumed he had again—but he refused to swallow the pills, repeatedly spitting them out in a slurry of chalky liquid. "I'll let you sleep after you take your medicine," I said, terribly frustrated. But, lying halfway on the bed, his feet on the floor, his arms crossed, my father said, "I am not going to take it."

He remained in bed all that day and night and then all day on Thursday and Friday. Muttering and moaning, he refused his meals. Harwinder managed to get him to swallow a few sips of mango nectar, but that was all.

By the time Rajiv and I got to the house after work on Friday evening, he hadn't eaten anything solid in two days. I tried to force him to eat some pudding or at least drink some Ensure, but the stuff just dribbled from his lips. "Why are you not hungry?" I demanded, beginning to feel panicked.

Harwinder answered for him. "He says people are sitting," she said. "They won't let him drink his tea."

When I called my father's primary care physician, Dr. Sandy Balwan, she asked me if I wanted to take him to the hospital emergency room. But my siblings and I had already decided against this. My father had been virtually bedbound for months, with little appetite, and he had been losing weight. He was dying, no doubt, and a hospital was the last place we wanted him to be.

Balwan suggested hospice care to help us look after him at home. Hospice would focus on my father's comfort; a nurse would deliver morphine and other medications to the house to help us manage his symptoms in his waning days. I immediately agreed. Though it was a Friday evening, Balwan said she would make some phone calls to see what she could arrange for the weekend. At the very least, she would expedite a referral to Hospice Care Network of New York for the following week.

Looking back, I am amazed at how quickly the decision for hospice got made. Most families, in my experience, will put off making the decision until a cycle or two of hospitalizations have passed. Like my father, I usually approach momentous decisions with ponderous deliberation (though, unlike me, after giving due consideration to a dilemma, he never vacillated). But that evening I made the decision for hospice right on the phone—without, in fact, even discussing it with my brother, though I knew he would agree. The groundwork for the decision had been laid over the previous six and a half years of witnessing my father's slow decline. Yet that Friday night, trying to force him to take in some nourishment by mouth, I could not wrap my head around what the choice would mean.

Since he'd been in bed for more than two days, Harwinder and I decided to take my father downstairs for a change of scenery. With some effort, we pulled him out of bed. His legs shook as he tentatively placed his feet on the carpet, and his hands trembled while gripping his walker. Somehow we managed to get him down the hallway to the stairs. "Put your hand on the wall," Harwinder instructed in Punjabi. "Now put the walker aside and hold the railing."

He struggled down the steps, pausing on each for a minute or more as we held him up. "Put your foot there," Harwinder directed. It was almost as if he had forgotten how to walk, how to move his legs in a coordinated fashion.

When he got to the bottom step and saw a jacket lying across his chair, he immediately said, "Whose coat?"

"That's Rajiv's," I said. "He is waiting for you."

My brother was lying on the leather couch, talking on the phone.

He stared at us blankly, not getting up to help, as if we were doing something wrong or stupid but he had decided not to say anything.

"He's stable . . ." I heard him say. "No, we have no idea what's going to happen . . . Yes, he looks better now than he did three hours ago."

Harwinder and I got my father into my mother's recliner, where I lifted his legs, pulled off his boxers, and slipped on clean pajamas while he groaned miserably. "Sit back and relax now," I said. "Harwinder will prepare some tea." But no sooner had we gotten him settled than he demanded to go back to bed. This time, his legs failed him completely, and my brother and I had to carry him up the stairs. Rajiv heaved up his legs while I slipped my hands under his armpits. We staggered down the hall back to the bedroom as my father cursed at us for our lack of respect.

"This is the last time we will ever take him downstairs," my brother said after we got him back into bed. It wasn't clear whether this was a prophecy or a command.

Sitting at the bedside, I tried to piece together what had happened over the previous five days. I'd taken him to House of Dosas only on Sunday afternoon. Had he contracted pneumonia in the rain? Could he have had a stroke? Had the subdural hematoma somehow expanded? Could he have Covid? As a physician as well as a son, I was desperate for an explanation.

My wife, Sonia, and our daughter, Pia, came by that evening. Sonia made my father a milkshake but failed to get him to drink any of it. "You used to have a house in Fargo with many trees, beautiful linden trees," she said, trying to get him to talk, but he was in a deep slumber. He woke up briefly only when Pia spoke to him. "She is . . . beautiful," he managed to say before closing his eyes again.

The lack of nourishment had clearly left him profoundly dehydrated. Perhaps that was the reason, I speculated, beginning to vacillate over the decision for hospice, that he had collapsed coming back up the stairs. "If water is the problem, you should give him IV," Harwinder suggested. Sonia, a doctor, agreed. "You guys are giving up too fast," she said. "Two liters of fluid and Dad is going to spring right up."

Though my brother did not agree, he nevertheless drove to his hospital to pick up an IV kit and a few bags of saline. While he was gone, I noticed he had placed my father's will, along with an assortment of other papers, on the dining table. In the pile was a letter my father had written to Rajiv in 2004 that spelled out my parents' wishes regarding end-of-life care. The letter read:

> When we are gone, which is of course a fact of life, you will have to take over. As I discussed with you before, I want to invest our money in the Jauhar Foundation for Social Upliftment. The Foundation's responsibility will be to help the poor and the downtrodden, mostly in India and some in this country (we already give to the homeless shelters here in Fargo).
>
> I will make certain that neither of us becomes a burden on you in any way. If I go first, your mom will not leave this home to live with any of the kids (though of course she will visit you). And if she happens to go first, then I will stay alone in this house till the end. This is our firm decision. Moreover, if we happen to get very sick, we would not want any extraordinary means to keep either of us alive. We want to live only if we have a meaningful life. This will all be spelt out. Yet, in old age, we or either one of us would like to see you more frequently. For whatever little we have done for you, all we want in return is one thing: happiness of our children and of course our grandchildren.

At the end of the letter, I noticed, both he and my mother had affixed their signatures.

When Rajiv returned from the hospital, he set aside his reservations about the IV and quickly went to work. He had always been good with his hands, much better than me. Growing up, he had been the tinkerer and I had been the thinker. First, he threw a sterile sheet over my father. Then he tore open the IV kit and spilled its contents onto the drape. His fingers started moving rapidly, opening packages of needles, drawing up a saline flush, arranging the instruments he was going to use with the meticulousness of a chef. When he was ready, he cleaned the back of my father's hand with antiseptic and injected it with a tiny bleb of lidocaine to numb it up. There was no indecision as he took a 22 gauge needle and poked it through the paper-thin skin while Harwinder and I held down my father's arms and legs, causing the unleashing of a torrent of muted screams. Patting the dehydrated vein with his fingertips, Rajiv moved the needle back and forth until a burst of maroon filled the barrel. When he removed the syringe, unusually dark red blood dribbled out the hub of the needle and onto the blue drape. After removing the needle, Rajiv connected the IV catheter to a long piece of plastic tubing attached to a bag of saline. My father quieted down. Then, holding the bag over his head, Rajiv squeezed it to push the salt water into my father's collapsed veins. Since we didn't have an IV pole, my brother tied the bag to the ceiling fan with some orange sewing thread.

When he was done and the fluid was flowing, he turned to me and said, "I never thought I would have to put an IV into my own dad."

A hospice nurse came to the house around ten o'clock that night. (The hospice network had accepted my father as a patient earlier in the evening.) After the nurse, Leah, took a quick peek at my sleeping father, Rajiv and I sat down with her at the dining table to sign some paperwork. On the intake form, my father's diagnosis was written as "end-stage dementia." I was put down as his primary caregiver. For enrollment purposes I signed a Medical Orders for Life-Sustaining Treatment (MOLST) form stating that no attempt should be made to resuscitate him in the event of cardiac or respiratory arrest.

I asked Leah how long my father could survive, assuming he did not recover enough to take in nourishment by mouth, on IV fluids alone. Astoundingly, she said it could be a few weeks or even up to two months.

"Two months without food?" I said in disbelief.

"Yes," she said. She'd taken care of several patients with dementia who had survived that long. "Of course, there might come a time when you decide you don't want to give him fluid anymore," she said.

Her words hung in the room for a few moments.

"Can the fluid hurt him?" I asked.

"No, but it can prolong the agony," my brother said before she could respond.

"So you don't agree with the IV?" she said to my brother.

"Absolutely not," Rajiv replied.

"But he isn't the only one making the decision," I quickly added.

"Yes, we want to decide things unanimously," Rajiv said through gritted teeth. "If one of us disagrees with pulling back, we are going to do what that person says." Though he didn't say so, a few years earlier his mother-in-law, diagnosed with a terminal blood disorder, had been hospitalized in an ICU for several weeks before her death. The traumatic experience had affected him deeply.

"I learned long ago that families break down over these issues," my brother continued quietly. "So we will go with the weakest link." Then he walked out of the room.

After the forms were signed and Leah left, Rajiv and I decided we would take turns spending the night with my father. I volunteered to take the first night, so after Rajiv went home, Harwinder and I got my father ready for the night. First, we had to change his diaper. By then, almost a liter of saline had run through the IV, and the diaper and bed sheets were soaked. We put down the head of the hospital bed and pulled him up. Next, we tipped him to one side, then the other, to remove his soiled shirt and the wet sheets from under him. "No, Bubby," he cried, weakly kicking at Harwinder as she tsk-tsked sadly, wiping down his groin like a baby's.

When we were finished changing him, my father seemed more alert.

"You must be tired," he said tenderly to Harwinder.

"Tired I am," she said affectionately.

"Oh, my little lady," he murmured, the way he used to with my mother, and a wave of nostalgia washed over me. Thinking of my parents as they had been, and what was now undoubtedly in store for my father, tightened my chest and brought tears to my eyes. He looked quizzically at me as I sat crying softly on the twin mattress on the floor by his bed. "Where will you go now?" he mumbled.

"Nowhere," I said, trying to compose myself. "I'll be here with you." I was finally going to spend the night with him, just as I had promised.

"Don't worry," he whispered, counseling me as he always had. "Things will work out."

"How do you know?" I said.

"Because . . . they always do," he replied.

Someone from hospice care rang the doorbell at around one in the morning to deliver a "comfort pack" of dissolvable morphine and the fast-acting anti-anxiety drug Ativan, as well as a medicine called atropine to dry up airway secretions. I immediately put three-fourths of a milligram of Ativan under my father's tongue and gently closed his mouth. He had been tossing and lightly moaning but now quickly fell asleep. As he snored, his dry lips curled up into a half smile. When she came in at around four o'clock to check on him, Harwinder said, "Let's hope he goes laughing."

Though I periodically kept getting up to check on him, he slept soundly until morning. At around nine o'clock I opened the curtains to give the room some light. Shaking him gently, I was able to wake him, but there was no change in his condition: he was still delirious and unable to stand on his own. With Harwinder's help, I was able to get him to the bathroom, where he managed to sit on the toilet to urinate. However, when we got him back to bed, he quickly collapsed again.

I noticed then that the IV catheter was clotted with blood and that the fluid had stopped running. It must have happened the previous night when I briefly unhooked the plastic tubing while we were changing his clothes. I connected a saline-filled syringe to the IV and tried to force out the clot, but it didn't move. I was sure that the IV was blown and we would have to put in another one, but when Rajiv came over with breakfast, he expertly flushed the line and got the fluid started again.

My father remained in bed all that day, Saturday, mostly sleeping, though he would sometimes wake up groaning as if in pain. He hadn't eaten more than a spoonful of pudding in five days. Nevertheless, he was alive. And the IV was still running.

As he endured through that day and the next, I began to have second thoughts about the palliative approach we'd decided on. He had walked, albeit tenuously, into House of Dosas only a week earlier. Now he was lying on his deathbed? It didn't make sense. Rajiv reminded me of our father's own words in the 2004 letter: that he didn't want extraordinary measures performed to keep him alive. But I didn't want to do anything extraordinary. Just continue the IV fluids and maybe try giving him some antibiotics.

How were we supposed to interpret the directive he had written almost twenty years earlier in the context of his situation today, I wondered. Obviously becoming bedbound was not an outcome he had desired, but the letter did not make clear what he was willing to have done if it became a reality. Moreover, did the letter reflect his current wishes? What was meaningful to him as a working scientist in 2004 was very different from what had become meaningful to him in the prior few months, when spending time with Harwinder or even eating a spoonful of pistachio kulfi had given him genuine pleasure. My siblings and I judged those things to be simple, childlike, somehow beneath him, but wasn't that just our hypercognitive prejudice?

On Sunday afternoon we made a call to my sister, who would be flying in that night with her family. Twenty-two months earlier we'd had a conversation weighing the pros and cons of surgery to drain my father's subdural hematoma. Now we were facing a similarly grave decision, though the consequences felt so much starker.

"If we weren't giving him IV fluids, it would have happened by now," Rajiv said. "He would have died on Friday. I'll do whatever you say, but continuing IV fluids doesn't make any goddamned sense to me. This is not what he wants."

"So what should we do?" I snapped. "Stop the fluid and give him morphine because we cannot deal with it anymore?"

"No, I won't allow that," Harwinder chimed in. She was sitting at her usual perch on the stairs, listening. "He is going to go: one day, two days, four days. But we are not going to make him dead with medicine."

"I am not saying we would do that—"

"And I won't let you do it," she said, interrupting me. "Even if he lies here for two months. If you don't want to give the IV fluid, don't give it. But we are not going to make him dead with medicine."

"It's not that we can't deal with it," Rajiv said to me, ignoring Harwinder. "It is a question of what he wants. He was very clear: no heroic measures."

"I don't want to do anything heroic! Give him antibiotics and fluid and, I don't know, maybe check blood and urine tests."

"But what are you trying to save him for?" my brother cried. "Last thing this man would ever want is to shit in his bed every day. I mean, he couldn't turn on the laptop, he couldn't put the phone to his ear. The man who wrote books would say, 'What the fuck are you doing?' I was in the room when Leah came on Friday. I had to walk out because I was so disgusted. You made me put in the IV. Now you want to do blood and urine tests?"

"I am not saying—"

"No, that's exactly what you're saying! You're doing what you usually do, the indecisiveness, the vacillation. You've written about this in *The New York Times*, for God's sake, not doing too much at the end of life. If Dad was alive, he would sit you down and shake you and say, 'Sandeep, what the hell are you doing?'"

"He never once said to me that he wanted to die," I put forward.

"Because he no longer had the capacity to voice that feeling," Rajiv shot back.

"So we are making this decision for him. He didn't—"

"He did! Years ago, when he wrote that letter."

"So we are following his wishes back then, not necessarily his wishes today."

"Isn't that what a health care proxy is supposed to do? Follow his wishes when he was of sound mind? All we have is those past conversations."

Of course I understood what he was saying, and later, when I was honest with myself, I recognized that in viewing our father, lying there, wearing a diaper, as the same man he'd once been— as still connected to the person he was when he wrote that letter—

my brother was in a way being more respectful of our father and his personhood than I was. Yet the fact that our father, having gone without nourishment for more than four days, was seemingly still fighting to live broke my heart. Who were we to decide that his life was no longer worth living and that it was his time to die when he himself had not made (or perhaps was incapable of making) that decision?

"I feel like he is saying, 'Help me out. Give me a fighting chance,'" I said.

"He is not saying that! He is at the level of a child. All he has is plus-minus: plus pain, minus pain. I have not wavered one minute. I told you that the dissenting opinion would decide. So if you want to draw blood and check his urine, I'll go along with it. But I totally disagree. This is not a life. This is not what he would want."

He asked Suneeta for her thoughts.

"We have to listen to what he said," my sister said, her voice breaking, "because that's what he would want. He wouldn't want what's happening right now, prolonging it for a week or two. We can't do that."

Rajiv again read aloud the letter my father had written: "'We would not want any extraordinary means to keep either of us alive. We want to live only if we have a meaningful life.'"

"You know, he had the ability even back then to have Mom sign the letter," Rajiv said. "I find that amazing. In my lifetime, he never had Mom sign a letter with him."

"So he was really adamant about this," Suneeta said. She began sobbing.

"Sun, it's okay," Rajiv said. "I was sad on Wednesday when I first saw him but I'm okay now. I'm like how I was with Mom. This is not him. This is not our dad." He turned to Harwinder. "What do you say?"

"What is there to say?" she replied after a pause. "Do what you want, but he has the same amount of time. Whatever is written in the books, that is how long he is going to live."

Suneeta flew in that evening with her husband and two children. Later that night we sat in my father's bedroom and told family stories while he slept. It was a way to celebrate him, but it felt like a kind of rehearsal, too, for the funeral. My brother shared memories from the three and a half years we lived in Wales: our house on Bow Street, the family picnics at Devil's Bridge. It was bittersweet to hear his recollections of a time when our family was whole, though I remembered some of them differently. The piano had been at the back of the house, not by the front door. My mother had been there when we got home from school. We'd watched *Tom and Jerry* in Kentucky, not Wales. And watching my father lying there, his body contorted, gulping air, it was hard to believe that he had ever chased us around the house for breaking the window in the front door.

I did not want to get out of bed on Monday morning. The previous few days had felt like a dream—or perhaps I just wished they had been a dream. But that morning I knew a great upheaval was coming, something I'd feared my whole life, and I did not want to face it.

Before I left my house, my sister texted me:

"The nurse is here. She said we need to give him both medicines, the morphine and the other one, EVERY FOUR HOURS. She said it's extremely important that we do that. She says that what we're giving him is not enough. He will not die unless he is at peace. She is increasing both dosages. Also she said get rid of the IV. She said we are prolonging his suffering by keeping in the IV."

When I arrived at the house, I immediately went up to the bedroom to check on my father. His mouth was open: a thick crust coated his lips and tongue. I discerned a flicker in his eyes when I said good morning. Even though he was semicomatose (because of the morphine or his underlying condition), he still seemed to sense my presence.

The hospice nurse, Jasmine, was in the room and asked me if we could talk. We sat down together at the bedside. Before she could say anything, I asked if it was still possible to make a change in my father's care plan. I wanted to know if we could still give him a trial of antibiotics and draw blood samples to try to understand what had happened.

My brother walked out of the room.

"We can certainly do that," Jasmine said softly. "I understand this is a very sudden change. I don't think it's going to bring him back, but we can do it if it will make you feel better." She asked me how my father's functioning had been before the downturn.

"It was bad," I admitted. He'd been eating less and having a harder time getting around. Still, he'd had lunch with me at a restaurant just a week earlier. "I don't feel like he's declaring that this is the end," I said uncertainly. "Maybe we could support him and give him a chance to rally from whatever has happened."

She thought for a moment. "What do you think he would want if he could participate in this conversation?" she asked.

"Which father?" I asked, distilling the conundrum I'd been struggling with into a question. "The father I knew when I was a boy would look at the father today and say, 'This is not what I want.' But the father from a month ago might say, 'Help me get through this so I can have a few more weeks or months.' I hear myself telling him, 'Dad, your life isn't meaningful,' and he says, 'Who are you to tell me this?'"

She nodded thoughtfully. I could tell she knew where she wanted me to go but did not want to rush me there.

"His blood pressure is still 130 over 80, and he hasn't eaten in over a week," I said. "He is fighting. It's very hard for me to look at that and not wonder if we should do more to support him."

"This is actually similar to the course we often see in our end-stage dementia patients," Jasmine replied. "It isn't uncommon for families to say that it was almost like a light switch. Their loved one went to bed one night and woke up the next day and suddenly what was normal wasn't normal anymore. Now, maybe something acute happened, like a urinary tract infection, that changed the trajectory of how quickly the changes were happening. But urinary infections *are a part of end-stage dementia*," she said slowly and emphatically.

I thought for about a minute about what she'd said. Till then, in my mind, my father's rapid slide had seemed somehow separate from the disease we'd been struggling with for almost seven years. But by framing it as a consequence of the disease to which we had already reconciled ourselves, the nurse suddenly made the decision not to treat more acceptable to me.

"I want him to die peacefully," I told her. "But right now it feels like we are trying to eke the death out of him."

"Remember, you didn't make your decisions in a bubble," she replied. "You didn't take someone who was healthy and decide not to offer him antibiotics and put him on morphine. His body showed you signs that it was already declining. But the process can take a lot longer than families anticipate. Your body can survive for a long time without food—especially if it is getting fluid," she added.

"So, what would you advise?" I said, knowing the answer.

"I would not recommend IV fluids at all," she answered firmly. "It sounds to me like your dad was trying to tell you guys that if his life ended up like this, to let him go."

We sat for a couple of minutes in silence.

My brother came in. "So what have you decided?" he said.

I looked over at him, at his tall-in-the-saddle confidence. We'd always had such different ways of dealing with problems. He'd never had much tolerance for indecision. As a caregiver with a surgeon's mentality, he knew what needed to be done, and I could tell he was finished waiting for me to figure it out.

I could only shake my head. "You decide," I said to him.

So he did. "Please take out the IV," my brother said to Jasmine before quickly leaving the room.

A person can survive without water for about three days. My father lasted four. Four endless days of us sitting at his bedside, playing bhajans, wordlessly waiting for the inevitable to happen. About a day after we took out the IV, he began to display "agonal" breathing—loud gulps of air that caught like cotton in his sticky airway, followed by prolonged periods of apnea, or no breathing—a pattern that frequently heralds death. As it intensified, we increased the dose of morphine. In my work with terminally ill heart failure patients, I have often encountered the doctrine of "double effect": that actions in the pursuit of a good end—for example, symptom relief—are morally acceptable even if they result in a negative outcome—such as death—as long as the negative outcome is unintended. Increasing the dose of my father's morphine, I'd been taught, was ethically justifiable if preventing suffering was the primary intention and hastening death was an inescapable side effect. Yet what exactly our intention was in those last few days still isn't clear to me.

"You can go, Dad," Rajiv whispered, but he wouldn't give up. A part of me had known he would do this; he'd always had such an incredible tolerance for suffering. "The more you wait for it, the longer God is going to make you wait," Harwinder admonished. Her comment made me remember what an elderly woman with terminal heart disease had once told me: "My husband always said the hardest thing to do is to die. I always thought it would be easy."

Watching him struggle to hold on, I thought about what a complicated man he had been. A loner who craved recognition. A decorated scientist with no small share of prejudices and biases. A "modern" thinker who relied on ancient aphorisms and clichés to guide him. The perplexing disease that finally did him in was no less a reflection of the man. For almost seven years his dementia had seemed undignified, a source of shame in our lives, a sort of pagan force. But deterioration, I realize, is part of the natural state of things. And so perhaps dementia, as an expression of our inevitable dissolution into disorder and decay, is not so foreign, unnatural, or inhuman after all.

He took his last breath on Friday morning. I'd planned to be at the house at eight o'clock, but I overslept. When I arrived at three minutes before nine, my sister frantically summoned me upstairs. "Dad, Sandeep is here," my brother loudly announced as I entered the room. I rushed over to the bedside and touched my father's stubbled cheek. He took a long breath and then, after about fifteen seconds, another one. Then he went silent. We waited for another breath as we had for almost four days, but it never came.

As he drifted away and people began to wail, I experienced a strange remembrance. It was from our second year in America. I was nine years old and learning to ride a bike on the sloping dirt hill behind our house in Kentucky. It was a cheap girl's bike that my father had bought on sale from Kmart. Built for a paved street, it made creaky metallic sounds as I coasted precariously down the furrowed trail.

As I used to remember it, when my father quickly realized that I could make it down the hill on my own, he lost interest and went inside. But that sunny March morning as I gripped his lifeless body, for some reason I saw him running beside me. I was pedaling furiously down the rutted path, flying over sticks and weeds as my father kept pace to make sure I did not fall. I know it didn't happen this way; I can't imagine that it did. But it is my memory now. I'll keep it.

ACKNOWLEDGMENTS

I am indebted to many people for their help and support during the writing of this book.

My agent, Todd Shuster, has been a friend and advocate for more than two decades. I am grateful for his faith in me as a writer.

I owe an enormous debt of gratitude to my brilliant editor, Alex Star. Alex's editorial acumen is present on every page of this book. I feel very fortunate to have worked with him.

I also want to thank several other colleagues at Farrar, Straus and Giroux: Alex's assistant, Ian Van Wye, for helping to edit the manuscript and for attending to so many important details during the course of this enterprise; Christina Nichols, copy editor extraordinaire; and my wonderful publicity team, headed by Lottchen Shivers. And of course I am indebted to FSG's publisher, Mitzi Angel, for giving me the chance to write the book in the first place.

I am lucky to work with a tremendous group of colleagues at Long Island Jewish Medical Center, including Maureen Hogan, Tamara Jansz, Patti Ursomanno, and Tracey Spruill, who supported me through this project. I also owe a special thanks to my chiefs, Rohan Bhansali and Jeff Kuvin.

Several other friends and assistants have earned my heartfelt appreciation, including Danielle Ofri, Daniella Cohen, Maureen Miller, Cody Elkhechen, Dee Luo, Morish Shah, Emily Lemieux, Zach Meyer, Dinesh Kommareddy, and my wonderful former editor, Paul Elie. They all critiqued early drafts of the manuscript or assisted me with research.

Of course, I am ultimately responsible for these contents. If there are any mistakes, the fault is mine and mine alone.

I save my deepest gratitude for my family: my wife, Sonia, and my dear siblings, Rajiv and Suneeta. My children, Mohan and Pia, were deep reservoirs of love and support throughout this enterprise. They are the twin lights of my life.

Finally, I am grateful to my father for all his pushing and prodding throughout my life. He was my first example of an author, and as much as I might not want to admit it, for good or bad, and in so many different ways, I am him.

INDEX

Page numbers in *italics* refer to photographs.

A NOTE ABOUT THE AUTHOR

Sandeep Jauhar is the bestselling author of three acclaimed books, *Intern*, *Doctored*, and *Heart: A History*, which was named a best book of 2018 by *Science Friday*, *The Mail on Sunday*, and the Los Angeles Public Library, and was a *PBS NewsHour / New York Times* book club pick; it was also a finalist for the 2019 Wellcome Book Prize. A practicing physician, Jauhar writes regularly for the opinion section of *The New York Times*. His TED Talk on the emotional heart was one of the ten most watched of 2019. To learn more about his work, follow him on Twitter: @sjauhar.